610.7306

Nursing Frontiers

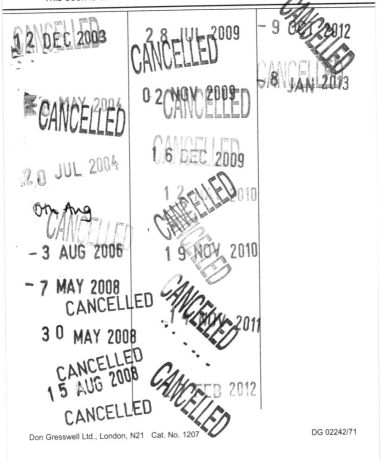

Dedication

This book is dedicated to my wife Ruth and our daughter Lara Róisín who arrived just as the book was going to print. I would therefore like to add a big 'thank you' to all the staff of the City Maternity Hospital, Carlisle!

Nursing Frontiers: Accountability and the Boundaries of Care

Mike Walsh, PhD BA(Hons) RGN PGCE DipN(London)

Reader in Nursing and Professor of Nursing Development
St Martin's College, Carlisle, UK

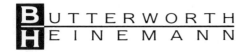

OXFORD   AUCKLAND   BOSTON   JOHANNESBURG   MELBOURNE   NEW DELHI

Butterworth-Heinemann
Linacre House, Jordan Hill, Oxford OX2 8DP
225 Wildwood Avenue, Woburn, MA 01801-2041
A division of Reed Educational and Professional Publishing Ltd

ℛ A member of the Reed Elsevier plc group

First published 2000

© Reed Educational and Professional Publishing Ltd 2000

Cover design and cartoons © Sarah Hough 2000

British Library Cataloguing in Publication Data
Walsh, Michael J.
  Nursing frontiers: accountability and the boundaries of care
  1. Nursing – Practice – Great Britain
  I. Title
  610.7'3

ISBN 0 7506 4316 1

Library of Congress Cataloguing in Publication Data
Walsh, Michael.
  Nursing frontiers: accountability and the boundaries of care/Michael Walsh.
    p. cm.
  Includes bibliographical references and index
  ISBN 0 7506 4316 1
  1. Nurse practitioners   2. Nursing – Practice.   I. Title

RT82.8.W35 2000
610.73–dc21   99–058096

Composition by Genesis Typesetting, Rochester, Kent
Printed and bound in Great Britain by Biddles Ltd, Guildford and King's Lynn

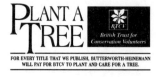

Contents

Preface

Time was away and somewhere else
The waiter did not come, the clock
Forgot them and the radio waltz
Came out like water from a rock
Time was away and somewhere else.

Louis Macneice. *Meeting Point (1941)*

These words convey to me a sense of time standing still. There are occasions in my nursing career when that same sensation still grips the heart and I feel, 'here we go again', struggling to move nursing practice forward. However comfortable it may be to stick to old familiar ways, this is not an option any more, we have to move on. This book is an attempt to tackle some of the key issues involved in moving nursing on, but doing so in such a way that nursing is in charge of its own destiny rather than dancing to the tune of others.

The book starts with reviewing just what we mean by 'caring' and challenges some taken for granted notions about nursing being a profession. It ranges over practical issues such as what the law and the UKCC have to say about expanding nursing practice before moving on to look at the growth of the Nurse Practitioner movement and the impact of both Nursing and Practice Development Units. The discussion continues with the exploration of an exciting new model for understanding change that has been developed by Alison Kitson and her collaborators at the RCN Institute. This stresses the importance of evidence, context and facilitation in the successful implementation of practice development

I have also thrown in some challenging new ideas from outside the mainstream of nursing which, I believe, shed valuable light upon the struggle to develop nursing practice. The work of Richard Dawkins on evolution has thrown up the notion of memes as an explanation of cultural evolution. Memes are replicating pieces of cognition that pass from one generation to the next in a way analogous with genes. They are the ideas and myths that sustain culture and can be remarkably persistent. This book suggests that an understanding of memes can go a long way to explaining the persistence of nursing rituals and the change-resistant nature of nursing. Nursing models, however, can be seen as failed memes as they lacked the ability to replicate themselves widely into the nursing meme pool. Memes can, however, be exploited in a positive way by those of us wanting to see sustainable development in nursing.

Nursing is about interconnectedness and a recognition that the whole is more than the sum of the parts. This finds an expression in the science of Complexity and Chaos theory. This book urges nurses to study these fascinating and rapidly growing areas of human intellectual activity, as many nursing and health care phenomena are more readily understood when thought of as examples of complexity in action. Boundaries between professions are reinterpreted in terms of chaos theory and this analysis leads to the deduction that boundaries cannot be expected to be clearly delineated 'lines in the sand'. There will always be grey zones of complexity at boundaries rather than neat lines. The importance of this lies in the fact that this is precisely where much practice development is taking place today, at the frontiers of nursing. Innovation and experimentation frequently take place at the outer boundaries of nursing where there is overlap with medicine and other professional groups. It is a mistake to try to squeeze such activity to one side or another of an artificial line. It is far more useful to accept the nurse practitioner for example as what he or she is, a new breed of practitioner whose roots are in nursing and who is working primarily in the best interest of the patient at all times. Such innovations should be welcomed rather than stifled by attempts at professional pigeon holing.

I hope you will find this a challenging read and that the book will set you off thinking in new ways about nursing. We need to recognize as a profession that the hands of the clock are turning, time has not stood still, and we need to move on.

CHAPTER 1

The rhetoric and reality of caring

Darling, this is goodbye. The words are
Ordinary but love is rare.
So let it go tenderly
As the sounds of violins into silence. . .
Let love go like a young bird flying from the nest

Kathleen Raine (1943), *Parting*

Introduction

Caring, emotion and love are interwoven and the words quoted above capture some of this relationship. In Kathleen Raine's words, although two people may be parting, the caring remains. Nurses care, but do they do so in a way that is different from love? Is there caring and professional caring? Can we divorce emotions from caring? These are some of the key questions that have led nurses to reassess the nature of their relationships with patients. The traditional approach of being cold, clinical and distant from patients associated with the dictum of 'never get too involved' has been questioned by a new, holistic approach which requires engagement with the patient as a person. Where does this leave caring in modern nursing?

Caring does lie at the heart of nursing; few would disagree with that proposition. The daunting volume of literature on the topic of caring unearthed by the trawl through the library which I undertook in preparing this chapter supports this view and I can well believe the results of a computer search by Judith Sadler who found 1801 references to papers on caring contained in the Cumulative Index of Nursing and Allied Health Literature in the 5-year period ending 1992 (Sadler, 1997). Caring therefore is the key concept around which nursing is constructed. The purpose of this introductory chapter is to try to make sense of this mass of words and explore what the theoreticians have said about caring in the light of research evidence about what happens in the real world. The oft stated and rather simplistic view that medicine is about cure while nursing is about care will be subjected to scrutiny in an attempt to show that things are not as black and white as they seem. A major theme running throughout this book is that of accountability and the analysis of caring undertaken in this chapter will inform that debate as the book unfolds. Take care and read on.

The concept of care

There is an Everest of literature on the concept of care and its application to nursing, some of which has a great deal in common with the summit of that famous mountain, i.e. lost in the clouds and surrounded by a highly rarefied atmosphere that few of us could survive in or make sense of. That does not prevent us admiring the beauty of the mountain and aspiring to scale its flanks, even if we do not reach the summit. So it is with caring; we need to know the shape and contours of the concept so that we will recognize it when we see it and as nurses we can only carry out our role, like the Sherpas, on that mountain. We need therefore to be able to get to grips with caring and understand what it means in the nursing context.

Much of the early literature on the subject of caring came from North America. The modern pioneer of caring as a fundamental component of nursing was Leininger who began writing seriously about the concept over 20 years ago and described it as the central and unique focus of nursing (Leininger, 1977, 1981). Caring is a subjective phenomenon which means different things to different people. Because of its subjectivity it is also context dependent which means that the relative importance of the various attributes that make up caring will change depending upon the situation in which the care is given. I care passionately about the football club that I have supported all my life (Manchester City) but in a different way from which I care for a patient in the A&E department. The context is different and so the meaning of the word 'care' is different.

The situation is complicated further as the words 'care' and 'caring' are often used interchangeably when they are not. Care can be a noun, the thing that is given, such as physical assistance to wash and dress, but it can also be a verb which involves interaction with another person; e.g. feeling for, being attentive to or valuing somebody (Sadler, 1997). There are two very different ideas contained in these meanings, as the former is essentially something physical or instrumental, while the latter is about emotion and communication. Care in this sense means that the nurse has to connect with the patient in a psychosocial way. The term 'caring' is the process of interaction between the patient and nurse which results in the delivery of care and which, as we have seen, can either be just attending to the physical needs of the patient or take on a deeper and more emotional meaning. In either sense caring is intentional, it is something the nurse does deliberately usually with some outcome in mind.

The association between psychosocial care and connection with the patient has been analysed by Wilde (1997). She considers that the process of connection requires good communication skills and intentionality on the part of the nurse. However, communication is a two-way street and for effective communication to occur, the patient has to be equally involved. A patient who is cognitively impaired, unconscious, does not speak English or just a poor communicator is going to be a challenge for the nurse, however good his or her communication skills. The road leading from good nurse/patient communication to nurse/patient connection and on to psychosocial care should not be assumed to be straightforward because if the patient has communication difficulties this will impair connection, leading to a more minimalist approach by the nurse which gets the physical tasks done, but that is all.

If connection is established, Wilde (1997) considers this will lead to a nurse–patient relationship which has depth, a sense of co-presence and transcendence beyond the moment. Wilde describes co-presence as connecting at a 'soul level' with the 'true-center' of the other person while citing the work of Montgomery (1992) to explain that transcendence involves experiencing self as part of a greater force than self with the goal of nursing being to connect rather than achieve. Other suggested consequences of connection include harmony, healing, enabling and diminishing vulnerability. The context is important in making sense of such statements as clearly in a busy environment with a rapid turnover such as A&E, day surgery or a coronary care unit, some of these outcomes are more relevant than others (e.g. diminished vulnerability and harmony). In other contexts such as palliative care or mental health nursing, other outcomes such as depth, enabling or co-presence are more relevant.

We are however starting to climb above the day to day foothills of care into a more rarefied atmosphere when some of these notions are introduced and there is a need to look and see whether there is any evidence to support such rhetoric. After all, where or what is your 'true center'? What is a 'soul level'? These are terms that are subjective, ill defined and probably alien to many nurses. They are therefore in need of more scrutiny under the harsh light of real practice and we will return to them later. Wilde, however, has offered us a key insight into caring by stating that connecting, the intentional acts which will create a bond or relationship with a patient, promotes caring. She also notes that it does not necessarily take a great deal of time to connect with patients, providing good communication takes place.

The different dimensions of caring discussed above were captured by Morse *et al.* (1990) in their theoretical account of the concept. To these writers caring involved affect (emotion, feelings), a moral ideal (e.g. UKCC Code of Conduct), nursing intervention (e.g. physical care or psychological support), interpersonal relationship (communication and connection) and the human state (a holistic perspective on what it is to be human). British nursing has traditionally tried to exclude feelings from the world of nursing but, without such feelings, the only dimension of care left is the physical and instrumental, the tasks of nursing. We have introduced the term holistic to mean a rounded view of the whole individual, but there is much more in this concept and we shall return to it later.

Building on the work of Morse *et al.* (1990), Sadler (1997) has carried out a thorough literature review and substantial periods of observation of nurse–patient interactions in a North American setting (medical surgical wards). This has led her to define caring in this way:

> Caring is an individually and socially defined creative process of using presence, described by practising nurses as multidimensional work, where a holistic connection is made with a person to meet a recognised need.

There are some very interesting ideas embedded within this view of nursing. It captures much of the literature and it will be useful to take out key phrases from this definition and examine them more carefully. This will provide a framework to analyse the complex and extensive literature on caring. I realize that this may leave me open to the charge of reductionism, however, it is my intention to show that the basic ideas can be put back together again to make a whole rather than just left lying around as individual thoughts and opinions. It is the failure to put the pieces back together or to see how they fit in the bigger picture that characterizes the reductionism that nurses find distasteful in the so-called 'medical model'!

'Individually and socially defined'

Sadler uses this term to mean 'as defined by the persons in the situation'. Caring is therefore a subjective phenomenon that will be different for different people in different circumstances and will depend upon the perceptions of both patient and nurse, but especially the patient. This opens up the interesting concept of empathy which has recently become a central tenet of nursing theory and education. The classic early definition of empathy stems from Carl Rogers (1957) who described it as seeing the client's world as if it were your own, without losing the 'as if' quality. Forty years on the concept has changed little as Olson and Hanchett (1997) define empathy as the accuracy of our perceptions of others. White (1997) stresses the emotional, understanding and perceiving aspects of the concept but importantly also reminds us that empathy needs to be expressed to be of any value. The patient needs to know we are perceiving things in the same way as he is, for this insight to be of any use. Olson and Hanchett (1997) call this 'nurse expressed empathy' and define it as the skill of understanding what a patient is saying and feeling and communicating this understanding verbally back to the patient. This leads to 'patient perceived empathy', the patient's feelings of being understood and accepted by the nurse.

The notion of empathy has gained credence in many areas outside nursing, including the hard-nosed world of big business. Charles Handy describes empathy as being an essential characteristic of what he calls Zeus-like organizations which depend heavily upon personal communication to operate. For Handy (1995) empathy requires affinity and trust but it also needs the ability to think like the other person. This raises some difficult questions. Can a nurse feel affinity for a patient when, for example, she is from a totally different ethnic background and may not even speak the nurse's own language, or he has a different sexual orientation from the nurse or if he is engaged in criminal and antisocial behaviour such as drug dealing or beating up his wife? Can a nurse think like the patient when the difference between the nurse and patient becomes wider and wider in terms of characteristics such as age, social background, life experience or state of health?

Empathy is multidimensional, subjective, illusive and therefore difficult to research. It can be seen as a way of being or as a skill that can be
learnt like any other. These are not the same thing and neither will they
manifest themselves in the same way in the caring process (Price and
Archbold, 1997). The natural dimension of empathy, the way of being, is
a gift that we are born with in varying degrees and which will mature and
grow with age and experience assisted by self-awareness. The mature
50-year-old nurse is therefore better placed to empathize than the 21-year-
old newly qualified staff nurse simply by virtue of life experience.
Maturity is a necessary but not sufficient condition for higher levels of
empathy because if that 50-year-old nurse lacks self-awareness, does not
reflect upon life and the lessons it can teach us, her ability to empathize
will be diminished. Communication and reflective skills can be learnt,
however, so that nurses can improve their empathy skills without
necessarily showing true empathy. The extent to which a fit and well
25-year-old woman (nurse) can really empathize with a 65-year-old man
(patient) suffering from terminal illness is limited. As Price and Archbold
(1997) point out, to expect nurses, particularly the younger members of
the profession, to empathize with *all* patients, given the complicated,
multidimensional and still poorly understood nature of the concept is
unrealistic. Olson (1995) makes the telling observation that while much
has been written espousing the value of empathy to nursing, there is little
documented evidence of its efficacy in practice. In other words, even if we
knew what it was, does it make a difference?

It is therefore worth looking at some of the research evidence that does
exist on the subject of empathy and we start with a recent British study by
Baillie (1996) which explored what the term meant to a small sample of
nine nurses working on three surgical wards. Baillie found that the nurses
were aware that it was a difficult term to understand but that most of
them distinguished sympathy from empathy. To these nurses empathy
meant understanding and they pointed out that to be sympathetic
towards someone required less understanding and less of a close
relationship than empathy. Empathy therefore required closeness (affinity
as Handy puts it), but a certain detachment was felt necessary for
professional care to be given. Research by Savage (1995) on two medical
surgical wards found that nurses who did get close to patients did not
experience the levels of stress that traditionally might have been
expected. Some nurses actually found support from patients in their close
relationships and those nurses working in the ward which was run on a
primary care basis linked empathy, being non-judgemental and understanding patient needs as crucial for good quality care. The staff on the
other ward studied by Savage, which did not use primary nursing, talked
much less about empathy, but still stressed the need for good communication with patients.

Interesting as these two studies are, they are qualitative, small scale and
therefore do not lead to any generalizable findings. Olson and Hanchett
(1997) have tried to look at the efficacy of empathy and their research
involved a sample of 70 RNs and 70 patients, again on medical surgical
wards, in the USA. The researchers used a series of psychometric testing
tools to test the following hypotheses:

❏ Nurse expressed empathy is negatively correlated with emotional distress on the part of patients, i.e. the more nurse expressed empathy there is, the less distressed patients will feel
❏ Nurse expressed empathy is positively correlated with patient perceived empathy
❏ Patient perceived empathy is negatively correlated with patient distress, i.e. the less patients feel the nurses are understanding them, the more distressed they will feel.

The research did indeed establish statistically significant moderate correlations between the variables as predicted. Here is firm evidence that patient distress is linked to nurse empathy. It has to be acknowledged, however, that this is only one study and various other factors would also have been influencing patient distress such as personality, social factors and diagnosis. The bigger the sample the more confident the researchers could be that empathy was the key variable at work in explaining variations in patient distress. These findings of course only apply to adult general surgical and medical wards in the USA. There need to be more studies in other clinical areas involving larger samples before the positive impact of nurse empathy upon patient care can be firmly established. The strictures of Price and Archbold (1997) to beware uncritical acceptance of empathy as a panacea for nurse–patient relationships are worth remembering for, as they caution, empathy alone may not be a practical fit for the demands of clinical practice.

'Recognition of need'

The key question here is how good are nurses at recognizing the needs of patients? The evidence in this area is not encouraging as recent research by Lauri et al. (1997) indicates. They cite some small scale studies which showed that nurses were not very good at estimating patient need before presenting the results of their work in Finland which looked at perceptions of need among 92 medical/surgical patients and the 60 nurses who delivered their care over the period they were hospitalized. Patient need was divided into the four key areas described by Yura and Walsh (1976) and which, according to these authors, are independent of culture. If this is correct, the validity of the work outside Finland is enhanced, however no evidence to support this claim was advanced. The four areas were:

❏ Vital functions (circulation, breathing, body temperature)
❏ Functional health status (sleep, nutrition, mobility, elimination)
❏ Reactions to functional health status (feelings, emotions, sexuality, coping etc.)
❏ Environment (information about care being administered).

This study found that the nurses underestimated patient needs in the first three categories but seriously overestimated need in the latter. There was therefore a major mismatch between patient and nurse perceptions concerning all aspects of need in this study. However, with such a small scale and unrepresentative sample, it is difficult to generalize these findings to nursing in general.

To digress for a moment, the problem of small scale and unrepresentative samples plagues nursing research at the moment. Nursing's fascination with qualitative research which, by definition, is not generalizable, compounds this problem. Lack of funding for major studies and the low credibility given to nursing research leads to this state of affairs which, in turn, leads to nursing research lacking credibility and not getting the funds it deserves. We have therefore a vicious circle that nursing must try to break out of. If nursing research involved samples of hundreds or even thousands, scattered over a range of environments, then at last we would have findings that could be generalized with some degree of confidence. Far too many nursing research papers conclude by stating that the study needs replicating with a larger sample. You will notice this problem cropping up repeatedly through the book as various research studies are cited, so I will refrain from repeating this 'cri de coeur' as I do not wish to bore you with repetition!

If we return to the issue of need, there is a lack of evidence that nurses and patients define and perceive need for care in the same way. What scant evidence there is suggests a lack of convergence in this important area. These findings are consistent with the mismatch that also exists between what aspects of caring are valued most by nurses and patients. McKenna (1993) found that patients valued the instrumental aspects more highly than nurses who were likely to rate the expressive content of their work more highly (listening, comforting etc.).

The obvious implication for nursing practice is that it is crucial for the nurse to try to find out what the patient's point of view might be and then to work with this in planning and delivering care, rather than assuming that as the nurse, you know what is best. Various nurse theorists such as Riehl have tried to incorporate this simple idea into their models of nursing under the banner of subjective interactionism (Walsh, 1997a).

'Creative process of using presence'

This phrase means that caring involves an artistic and creative process and it also implies that the nurse uses self as an instrument and is fully present to the patient. Nursing needs to be a creative process if we recognize each patient as an individual with needs unique to that individual. Simply following standardized procedures in the traditional task-oriented way is no longer acceptable as care. We have to create care tailored to the needs of the person in receipt of that care.

There is a major shift in methods of planning care away from the nursing process and towards increasing use of protocols and critical pathways. The nursing process has largely failed to deliver individualized care and has consumed large amounts of precious nursing time filling in forms (Walsh, 1997b). The critical pathway concept makes use of the fact that a significant proportion of care required by patients with a similar medical condition is similar and therefore amenable to preplanning and measurement against set standards. The result is that a great deal of nursing time is saved and there exists a potentially very powerful quality assurance mechanism. The danger, however, is that too much emphasis is placed on slavishly following a preplanned pathway of care, regardless of individual need. Nurses working with critical pathways therefore need to be sure that there is sufficient flexibility for creative solutions to individual problems if they are to remain true to the principles of care.

For most of the 20th century nursing has lived in the shadows of medicine. Within medicine the prevailing paradigm has been the scientific one and this has served medicine well on many counts. Nursing has therefore followed in the footsteps of 'the men in white lab coats' and most nurses today have an educational background that owes more to the medical sciences than the psychosocial disciplines. The end of the century has, however, seen a major shift away from the scientific paradigm as the belief that scientific and technological rationality would solve all our problems has been shown to be unfounded. This modern belief has therefore given way to what is known as post-modernism; different ways of trying to find new explanations and meanings in life.

This presupposes that there is a meaning to life of course, for it may just be that the universe we observe is the universe of the eminent evolutionary biologist Richard Dawkins, who has written of the indifference of nature; this universe consists only of electrons and selfish genes replicating themselves with various degrees of success in accordance with Darwinian principles. This universe '. . . has no design, no purpose, no evil and no good, nothing but blind pitiless indifference.' Life is all about DNA and as Dawkins puts it; 'DNA neither cares nor knows. DNA just is. And we dance to its music' (Dawkins, 1995 p.155). This bleak view of life and the universe is cold comfort and not surprisingly many people find it hard to accept, despite the impeccable science that underpins it. Those who would dismiss science as having failed might also reflect on how they would be able to read this book in the dark without the science and technology to generate electricity and hence light. They might reflect upon the failings of science and reductionism as they fly at 30 000 feet in a modern jet on their way to their latest international conference. As Cohen and Stewart (1994) point out, it is precisely those laws and scientific discoveries that they reject which allows that jet to fly safely to its destination. In looking at the views of eminent American nurse theoreticians such as Jean Watson, it is worth remembering that the post-modernist rejection of scientific rationality is open to such challenges!

Watson (1997) writes that reality and truth are no longer objectively defined while connecting with each other and the universe in the cause of creating wholeness becomes part of the new reality and truth. Watson sees post-modernism as crucial to understanding what she describes as the re-emergence of the caring arts at the end of the 20th century. This rebirth is a counterpoint to what she calls the isolation, detached treatments and sterile technology of modern health care. The artistry of caring is said to draw from the human encounter, it is about engaging and connecting with people. Watson has a point when she describes modern health care in these terms, as much of it has become very high-tech, losing the human element in the process. She is also right to stress the interpersonal nature of caring. Unfortunately her views on caring then take on a rather more esoteric perspective:

> A caring moment is art serving all at once, connecting an individual spirit with the universal, art serving as mediator between matter and spirit. . . Caring and the arts touch the human soul which calls forth the continually mysterious emergence of beauty and spirit from matter.'

It is doubtful that many patients would recognize caring in these terms. Experience suggests that few nurses would either. Theoreticians who wax lyrical with such vaguely mystical language are losing touch with the real world in which most patients and nurses live. Unless their writings reflect reality and are accessible to nurses, they will have little influence on practice and the important messages contained in their writings will be lost in the hyperbole and psychobabble of New Age mysticism. Nurses also have to be politically realistic and recognize that power and resources in the health care system do not lie with people who speak this kind of language.

The notion of presence requires the nurse to recognize that simply being with a patient can be therapeutic in itself and therefore the nurse is a therapeutic tool. Henson (1997) writes of mutuality as a mode of relating that involves the patient and nurse in working towards mutually agreed goals leading to a respectful interrelationship, which it is suggested works well in stressful situations. The nurse presences him- or herself alongside the patient in this view and by a process of exchange with the patient allows the patient to achieve beneficial outcomes. This does not mean swapping equivalent stories. The patient may explain that he is feeling anxious about losing his job, mutuality does not mean telling the story of how the nurse once lost her job and took up nursing as a career move which was the best thing she ever did! Mutuality, according to Henson, is about exchanging things which are different but which balance so, in the above example, the nurse exchanges the patient's story for a discussion about alternative careers the patient may follow. The intention is to cancel out the anxiety and distress the patient is feeling with a problem-focused coping strategy. Mutuality therefore lies at the midpoint in a continuum stretching from paternalism to autonomy, telling the patient what to do on the one hand or reminding him he is free to do what he likes and walking away on the other. Above all mutuality requires respect, unlike collaboration which may not involve equal participation.

This idea of the nurse and patient involved in an exchange is not new. Morrison and Burnard (1997) cite this as one of the main reasons why nurses care about patients. They refer to the earlier work of Homans (1961), who wrote that the open secret of human exchange is to give to the other person something that is more valuable to him than it is costly to you and to get from him something that is more valuable to you than it is costly to him. Life is therefore a series of such interpersonal transactions. You may wish to reflect upon this notion in the context of your everyday working life in nursing. The care you give to a patient is more valuable to that person than it is costly to you to give. This is worth remembering when you have a patient you do not find it easy to get along with. Perhaps the reason you find this patient difficult is that the cost to you to give the care seems more than the value the patient places upon the care you have given. Conversely, the satisfaction you derive from caring for an appreciative patient who is making progress means you are getting more from the relationship than it is costing the patient to give.

Morrison and Burnard also remind us that one of the main ethical foundations of care is derived from the categorical imperative of Kant, that our behaviour should always be such as to illustrate a universal law, so that if something is right it is universally right. Caring is one such example. The reader should pause to reflect back on the views of Watson (1997) and the post-modernists who deny absolute reality and objectivity. This means that all things are relative and is at odds with Kant's universal imperative. This is a dangerous school of thought because it implies that caring is a relative concept and that therefore there are situations when we can care less than others or care not at all. That is hardly a sound ethical foundation for nursing (or medicine either!).

The phrase 'using presence' is worthy of further attention as presence means more than being physically present in the same room as the patient. Benner and Wrubel (1989) have expanded this concept to mean being available to understand as well as being with someone. The nurse is therefore not, cognitively speaking, standing apart from the patient, but rather is trying to understand the lived experience of that person's illness by sharing the humanity that characterizes both patient and nurse. This understanding or empathy requires the nurse to pay attention to the person who is the patient, not only in terms of what they are saying but also how they are saying it. It is also important to pay attention to what they are not saying and also their non-verbal communication at the same time. Only in this way can the nurse understand what Benner calls the 'situated meaning' experienced by the patient; in other words how things look to the patient which may be very different to how the nurse as an outsider sees things. Only by presencing, being accessible to the patient and letting the patient know this, can a degree of empathy be achieved which might allow the nurse to see the situated meanings with which the patient is working. It is easy to dismiss patient expectations as unrealistic, for example, because that is how they look to us; trying to see it from the patient's point of view might help avoid this error.

Multidimensional work

This phrase recognizes that the patient has physical, psychological, social, emotional and spiritual needs which the nurse is required to meet in order that care is delivered. For too many years nursing education in the UK concentrated only on the physical needs of patients to the exclusion of all others. The author is a product of that kind of training and I freely admit to the sense of amazement and understanding that suddenly came with the study of the social sciences a few years after I qualified. The London University Diploma in Nursing opened up a whole new world which suddenly allowed me to make sense of so much that had seemed incomprehensible before, simply because I gained some insights into aspects of human behaviour beyond the purely physical. Beware the siren call of the 'good old days' from those who would turn the nursing education clock back to the 1970s; they were the bad old days (and nights) so far as education was concerned because they only presented a unidimensional view of patient care and ignored the complex interplay of the social, psychological, emotional and spiritual aspects of the person. As Tuck (1998) points out nursing is not purely physical (nor purely psychological), despite the emphasis on the physical side of care which can be traced back to Nightingale.

The key question that has to be asked is whether nurses share this multidimensional view of care advocated by many leading nurse authors and which underpins the educational work of the National Boards in the UK? A useful step in answering this question comes from the work of Watson and Lea (1997) who have developed, from the caring literature, a tool which can be used to see how much relative importance nurses attach to the physical and more traditional technical aspects to care, compared to the psychosocial dimensions of care. Their tool (the Caring Dimensions Inventory) has been subjected to extensive development and piloting work in Scotland involving responses from 1430 nurses (response rate 47%).

Initial findings were promising in that the most highly rated aspect of care was listening to a patient followed by providing privacy, giving reassurance about a clinical procedure, and getting to know the patient as a person. Least caring activities were sharing your personal problems with a patient and feeling sorry for a patient. This suggests these nurses were aware of the difference between empathy and sympathy. Significant differences in the relative importance attached to psychosocial versus physical care did emerge, however. The older nurses were found to place greater emphasis on the physical aspects of care, which is consistent with the traditional approach to training and which identifies an issue for continuing education to address. The other statistically significant difference was that men placed relatively more emphasis on the psychosocial aspects of care than women. Men appearing more sensitive and supportive than women might seem surprising given the normal sexual stereotypes that place women in that role. This might be explained in terms of self-selection in that the sort of man who becomes a nurse is a more supportive person compared to the general population. However, MacDougal rightly reminds us of the disproportionate numbers of men in nursing management whom he suggests are operating within a traditional masculine framework of seeking power over others and who may have deliberately suppressed the more caring side of their nature in order to achieve these positions. Alternatively it may be that the men in the study were concentrated in the younger age ranges who showed higher levels of psychosocial awareness, while older men had gravitated away from clinical nursing into management and taken their different views of caring out of the study altogether.

The CDI is therefore a valuable tool which can allow us to explore how different groups of nurses see caring. Research by the author with the CDI revealed that a sample of nurses who had completed or were well advanced on the Royal College of Nursing Institute BSc Nurse Practitioner course (*n*=93) also perceived the psychosocial dimensions of care as significantly more important than a similar group of nurses (*n*=108) undertaking other level 2/3 post-registration courses. This contradicts assertions to the effect that nurse practitioners are only physicians' assistants who work with a medical model of care and suggests they have a more rounded view of care than traditional nurses.

Research evidence supporting the importance of seeing more than the physical aspect of care even in the most high-tech environments where patients' are critically ill comes from a study by Jenny and Logan (1996). Interviews with patients revealed that to them, caring was as much about the nurse's attitude as the nurse's actions. Phrases such as, 'Making me feel human' and, 'Making me feel like a person', summarized many of the patients' views about what makes a caring nurse in a critical care area. As Jenny and Logan state, caring involves maintaining a patient's personhood which clearly involves their psychological, emotional and spiritual well-being as well as their fluid balance and blood pressure. There are obvious links to Benner and Wrubel's view that nursing care involves an understanding of the lived experience of illness, for only in that way can the patient in the ICU bed be treated as a person. The patients' stories suggested that sources of distress were equally likely to be perceptions of an altered self as well as physical discomfort, once again underlining the importance of working for the whole person not just physical systems.

Uncaring nurses according to Jenny and Logan (1996) were described as impersonal and exhibiting only task-centred behaviour. This corresponds to what Benner and Wrubel describe as 'non-caring', i.e. being physically present only to get the job done rather than *being with* the patient, resulting in patients becoming dehumanized, fearful and even angry. The nurse acting as a humanizing agent in the increasingly inhumane high-tech hospital environment is a key theme emerging from the literature of the late 1990s (see Watson's views, p.9). Nurses have to remember that we are more than technicians and perhaps it is the ability to engage and understand patients undergoing often complex and invasive medical procedures that differentiates between nurses and technicians. The medical profession can decide for themselves on which side of this particular fence they wish to sit!

A holistic connection

Much has been written about holism in nursing. It is a reaction to the medical reductionism that breaks individuals down into separate systems and parts. Griffin (1993) suggests holism stands for harmony, which is something that we value, and it also contributes to our individual autonomy as a person. She rightly suggests that it translates in nursing terms into a respect for persons, openness, reflection and seeing situations comprehensively. It therefore has many of the characteristics of what Benner calls proficient nursing practice (Benner, 1984). However, when Griffin goes on to say that holism involves synthesizing the parts to make the whole and then rejects science and technology on the grounds that they are only reductionist, she is falling into the trap that we have already mentioned on p. 4, i.e. she is ignoring the fact that science works. It may not have all the answers at present, but a moment's reflection on your surroundings as you read this should reveal that without science and technology you would be in a very different and less welcoming environment. Try to imagine health care without modern technology and the science that underpins it and you will see what I mean.

The simple definition of holism given by Griffin (synthesizing the parts to make the whole), also exposes a weakness in the limited concept of holism, i.e. it does not take into account the context within which the whole exists (Cohen and Stewart, 1994). Breaking the individual down into subsystems is reductionist, but so long as the pieces of the jigsaw are reassembled to make the whole person, this is holistic. However, on its own that is not enough, for we have to understand the context within which the person lives in order to give meaningful care.

The importance of seeing the whole person is emphasized by Dahlberg (1996), who has written that the essence of health care is that it is something that happens between two people. The person giving the care (nurse) helps the cared for person to 'be' and 'stay as' a person despite the challenges to personhood presented by both illness and modern high-tech treatment modalities. Caring keeps alive our humanity and prevents the patient being reduced to an object. This theme has already been discussed (p. 2). Dahlberg's Swedish perspective emphasizes that care has to take place between two people not between two roles or stereotypes. In this way there is a 'true and meaningful meeting' which allows the nurse to see the person within the patient, but it requires the nurse to be a person and not retreat behind the professional defences we erect around ourselves when we go into role of nurses. The aim is open interpersonal communication between two people so that caring becomes dialogue.

True dialogue in this way is of course unpredictable for, as Pylkkanen (1989) describes it, dialogue is like the flow of a river between its banks; each influences the other in unpredictable ways at times and the banks of a river can never be relied upon to contain the river all the time. Floods may overtop the banks, erosion diverts the course of the river, slowing waters silt up the stream bed, water and banks constantly interact just as two people do in dialogue. Sometimes the person who is the patient will overflow the banks emotionally while the nurse may unintentionally divert the flow of conversation away from where the patient wants to go. Caring which involves really close dialogue with the patient as a genuine partner therefore contains this element of unpredictability, as the nurse is not exercising control in the traditional way. This also requires time and it is likely that one of the reasons for the success of nurse practitioner consultations with patients is that there is much more time allocated than in the usual GP consultation. The nurse practitioner may also be exercising less control over the conversation than a doctor traditionally would, thereby encouraging dialogue.

The nurse must, however, be honest with him- or herself and have knowledge of self derived from self-awareness and critical reflection, otherwise Dahlberg asserts the role of caregiver is a disguise and is used as a defence against perceived threats to the self. This implies that the caregiver needs a supportive environment within which to work; caring for the carer is crucial for caregiving. In common with the North American writers referred to above, Dahlberg agrees that the uncaring nurse is cold, emotionless and impersonal. Such a nurse denies the confirmation of worth of the individual patient and emotionally excludes them leading to fear and anxiety.

Holism therefore can be seen as a very useful concept, but it does have its limitations. It confirms and reinforces the notion that caring is multidimensional work involving much more than just seeing to a person's physical needs by carrying out a series of tasks. Seeing the patient as a whole person is, however, of little value if the nurse does not see him- or herself as a whole person also, rather than hiding behind a stereotypical nursing role. That is a risky thing to do sometimes, but we can only really care for another human being by being human ourselves. Holism as a concept views the whole unit under examination but does not necessarily place it in context. In espousing a holistic view of a patient therefore we must place that person and the care they require in the wider context.

To meet a recognized need

The final part of the definition emphasizes the importance of recognizing the patient's need for care. We have already seen that there is research suggesting nurses are not very good at this key area of care as Lauri *et al.* (1997) showed that nurses underestimated patient need in a wide range of areas including emotional support, sleep, nutrition and relationships. This study was carried out in Finland, however, and whether it is possible to apply these findings to the UK is open to debate.

There is evidence that nurses and patients do not place the same value on differing aspects of care. McKenna (1993) found that patients saw the more instrumental aspects of care as being more important than nurses did, while nurses placed greater value on the expressive emotional dimension. McKenna suggests this is because nurses take the instrumental aspects of nursing for granted. Whatever the explanation, it is not surprising that two groups of people looking at the same thing (nursing care) from different points of view will see it differently. This idea is developed further by Ovretveit (1992) who has analysed the quality of health care into three dimensions:

❏ Professional quality; what the nurse sees as important, e.g. drugs safely administered
❏ Client quality; what the patient thinks is important, e.g. food that is served hot
❏ Managerial quality; the sort of things that management consider important such as cost effectiveness.

This analysis reminds us that patients' perceptions of their needs are likely to be different from our perception. If we are therefore to achieve quality health care we must actively seek out the patient's needs rather than assume that as qualified nurses, we know best.

Much has been written about the issue of whether nurses intuitively know what patients need. Benner raised this issue in 1984 in her seminal work *From Novice to Expert* and it has remained a topic of much debate ever since. A splendid debate ensued in the UK literature with English (1993) opening the attack on Benner's notions of intuition which led Darbyshire (1994) to spring to her defence, championing the cause of intuition and claiming that the knowing was in the doing. Cash (1995) waded into the debate pointing out that if nursing knowledge was so subjective and could be justified solely by expert opinion intuitively knowing what was right, this would obstruct the development of nursing as it 'retreats into the validation of practice by authority and tradition'. A serious weakness in the 'intuitive knowing' argument has been highlighted by Walsh (1997a) who pointed out that in this era of evidence-based practice and professional accountability, a nurse called upon to justify any particular action in a court of law would be on very unsafe ground if he or she fell back upon intuition as the justification for actions taken. In fulfilling the legal duty of care that we owe our patients, we need a more tangible justification for care than intuition.

It may be that what is happening in so called 'intuitive practice' is that the expert nurse is drawing upon a wealth of experience and lessons learnt in practice in such a way as to be unaware of any logical problem solving mechanism. The holistic nature of nursing makes expert nurses very good at seeing the big picture and also at pattern recognition, whereas the more fragmented medical approach lacks this quality. Consequently nurses see when things are not fitting the pattern they should and can process knowledge and decision making skills so quickly that they are not even consciously aware of their cognitive processes. The result to an outsider looks 'intuitive'; 'How did she know that?' is a not uncommon response, but the apparently intuitive intervention was merely the result of experience, learning from that experience, pattern recognition, the ability to see the patient holistically and rapid decision making skills. Brilliant yes, intuitive no!

Putting the pieces back together

The definition of care offered by Sadler (1997) has served as a useful framework to analyse the caring literature. The key elements that emerge are:

❑ Caring is context dependent. The patient's environment will always have an effect upon the care that can be offered whether it be by the nurse, family, friend or others
❑ Caring ultimately is a one to one, interpersonal interaction. You have to recognize the person in the patient and in yourself, to really give care

❏ Caring is about being involved and having things matter. It is not about performing a series of tasks in a cold, detached fashion while thinking of other things

❏ Caring involves consideration of the person's emotional and psychological needs and the social circumstances in which they live

❏ Caring is about seeing things from the patient's point of view

❏ Caring is universal and to be cared for is a fundamental human right. It is a moral imperative which the professional nurse has to discharge equally for all, each according to his or her assessed need.

These are general principles which may be arrived at from an analysis of the literature. I offer no apologies for this reductionist approach as attempting to reduce complexity to simplicity offers a better opportunity for understanding than the impenetrable fog of jargon generated by some North American theorists. The key is that these principles are all consistent with each other and with the UKCC *Code of Professional Conduct*. It is therefore possible to integrate them into your everyday work, whatever clinical area you work in and, as a result, practise nursing that is genuinely caring. It is putting the pieces back together that allows us to avoid the trap of rampant reductionism and therefore lets us get on with the complex business of caring for people rather than diseases.

Problems with the practice of caring

The first part of this chapter has concentrated upon what nursing care should be. This is known as 'espoused theory' which Argyris and Schon (1974) define as our stated purpose or intention. Espoused theory is what we claim to believe in if asked; it is the way things should be. However, Argyris and Schon also pointed out that there is something called 'theory in use' which is what actually happens when we attempt to put our stated purpose into action. This may look very different from the espoused theory. This notion is familiar to nurses as the 'theory–practice gap'. It is therefore necessary to look at caring in action and see to what extent the practice of care by nurses measures up to the ideals expressed in the literature.

One of the early classic pieces of nursing research in the UK explored the notion of the 'unpopular patient' (Stockwell, 1972). This famous study showed that nurses labelled certain patients as difficult or unpopular which logically suggests the care they received was less than optimal. Patients who wanted more care than the nurse thought they should receive were called demanding and hence became unpopular. So too were patients who did not cooperate fully with care offered but, instead, exerted their own right to say 'no' or who argued about and questioned care. Another unpopular group were patients who were perceived as not belonging to the ward they were on or who had no right to be on the ward. This often meant patients admitted to a ward because the one to which they should have gone was full. Given the current near permanent bed crisis in many hospitals, it is possible that this phenomenon still exists today. The notion of the 'inappropriate attender' in Accident and Emergency departments again stems from the idea that the patient has no right to be there. Rather than seeing the services provided as inappropriate for the needs of the patient, doctors and nurses still blame the patient for being there and label him/her as an inappropriate attender, despite the research evidence to the contrary. These disturbing findings about general hospitals in the 1970s sat alongside a series of scandals involving patient abuse in some of the large mental hospitals at that time, creating a distinctly uncaring picture.

A quarter of a century later it is tempting to think that these findings relate only to the bad old days. Those who talk of the 'good old days' of matrons and traditional nurse training should reflect on what really happened in bygone times rather than viewing the past through nostalgia-tinted spectacles. However, there is ample evidence, even today, that some nurses still fail to care. For example, a study by Carveth (1995) showed that while all patients received equal *quantities* of care, those rated as 'difficult' received less care of a supportive nature than other patients. Fletcher (1997) raised several very uncomfortable issues starting with the issue of how nurses behave towards each other. We have already referred to the need to 'care for the carers', yet Fletcher reminds us of the hostility in clinical areas faced by many undergraduate and Diploma in Higher Education (P2000) students. Some registered nurses were frequently hostile and unwelcoming towards such students and were also guilty of demeaning and exploiting enrolled nurses. Fletcher also asks the uncomfortable question of how much actual care is provided by registered nurses as opposed to health care assistants, students and family members? Is it more accurate to talk of nursing not so much as the caring profession but as the 'answering the phone, going to meetings, arranging the off duty, chasing after doctors etc.' profession?

A further problem with the pressure of work that nurses find themselves under and the emphasis on health care outcomes, is that the focus of attention is on performing instrumental tasks in order to achieve high levels of patient throughput. Areas such as day surgery, outpatients, the health centre treatment room and the A&E department all suffer from the problem of needing to process high volumes of patients. Fletcher considers that the expressive or emotional aspect of care is sacrificed as a result and therefore, in view of the discussion in the first part of this chapter, we might suggest that the nursing offered to patients in such an environment is *uncaring* even though essential tasks are performed.

Evidence to support this suggestion is found in the work of Byrne and Heyman (1997) who looked at how nurses perceived patients in two busy A&E departments. They found that ambulant patients (the 'walking wounded') were perceived less favourably than those seriously ill or injured. The nurses were keen to work with these latter patients but were often dismissive or even rude about ambulatory patients. They also assumed that the more ill patients would have higher anxiety levels and therefore need psychological support, unlike the ambulatory patients who only received task-focused care. Research by the author (Walsh, 1993) showed that ambulatory patients can have very high levels of pain and anxiety in A&E which would not be met by a task-focused approach. Byrne and Heyman saw A&E nurses as working under a great deal of pressure and operating within a culture dedicated to getting on with the work and pushing the patients through the department as fast as possible. Talking to patients was seen as a luxury even though nurses recognized the importance of psychosocial care. The research did not, however, address the issue of aggression and violence directed towards A&E nurses which is becoming more widespread and may well be contributing towards an increased distancing from patients.

The problem of labelling and therefore stigmatizing patients, first highlighted by Stockwell (1972), is very much a live issue today, especially in regard of sexuality. Hayter (1996) has pointed out that as someone's sexuality is an integral part of that person, then any caring interpersonal relationship must take that into account. However, he points out that gay and bisexual people are being stigmatized by nurses and the negative attitudes associated with this process do adversely affect care. Hayter also notes that this problem has been exacerbated by AIDS. The result is emotional exclusion for gay and bisexual patients. The instrumental aspects of care are delivered, the jobs are done, but it is caring in one dimension only as the interpersonal aspects of care are omitted. The patient feels devalued as the nurse's attitudes manifest themselves particularly through non-verbal communication channels.

There are significant other sections of society who also feel prone to being stereotyped and patronized such as the elderly, the disabled and also people from ethnic minorities. The under-representation of ethnic minority groups is a major problem for all the public services such as the police, fire brigade, the teaching profession and of course, nursing. The NHS has been accused of having institutional racism embedded deeply within it and nurses have much work to do to treat people from ethnic minority groups as individuals not racial stereotypes. Educationalists have a major contribution to make to such a campaign but can easily fall into the trap of teaching stereotypes rather than educating nurses to value difference and variety alongside respect for other cultures and religions. This comment has equal validity with regard to education aimed at improving the understanding of other groups such as disabled or elderly people.

Ethically we know that nursing care should be allocated only according to need. As Olson (1997) points out, a caring concern for the patient as a person is not *part of* the treatment, it is *the reason for* the treatment. Olson, however, is able to cite evidence showing that if the nurse perceives the patient to be responsible for his or her own clinical situation, this adversely affects the quality of care delivered. He went on to demonstrate this effect by giving a sample of 51 RNs a series of five patient vignettes (short stories or case studies) and then subsequently interviewing them about the patients. The data showed a substantial proportion of the nurses believed that their sense of caring concern for the patient and hence the nature of their relationship with the patient, was adversely affected by the degree of responsibility that they attributed to the patient for the illness. It is as if the nurses were blaming the patient for being ill and, as a result, feeling that they had less obligation to deliver full interpersonal care. There are echoes of Stockwell's (1972) work in this study and reflection upon the reception often afforded a patient who has taken an overdose of drugs in a deliberate self-harm episode should make the reader realize that this phenomenon is still recognizable in the NHS today.

Olson's work raises the issue of attribution theory which is a key area of social psychology. The fundamental distinction in the attributions we make about other people's actions lies between internal and external attributions. An internal attribution means that we believe the reason for a person's apparent behaviour is located within the person rather than in outside circumstances (external attribution). There is a natural bias towards making internal rather than external attributions, so much so that it is sometimes called the fundamental attribution error. Nurses need to be aware of this natural bias as they strive to achieve the non-judgemental perspective that is necessary if care is to be delivered only according to need.

Attribution theory can also shed light on another aspect of nursing care. Using attribution theory, Meurier *et al.* (1998) hypothesized that if a nurse made an error that had serious consequences, he or she would be more likely to blame outside circumstances for the error rather than him/herself, i.e. an external rather than an internal attribution would be made. In simple terms we like to take the credit for success but blame others when things go wrong. This is a self-defence mechanism which helps preserve our sense of self-worth. However, making external attributions when things do go wrong is not conducive to learning from events, i.e. being a reflective practitioner.

Meurier *et al.* tested this hypothesis in a study involving 60 registered nurses (average time since registration 11.6 years). Each was given a hypothetical scenario involving a patient who had had prostatic surgery and who postoperatively had a urinary catheter which had to be secured to prevent dislodgement. The scenario continued with the catheter becoming dislodged and half the group were told this only had minor consequences but the other half were told it led to serious bleeding and greatly harmed the patient's well-being. The nurses were then presented with a questionnaire which explored responsibility and blame.

There were few differences between the two scenarios in terms of internal/external attributions, both groups tended to attach an internal attribution to the error, blaming themselves rather than the environment. This is at odds with what would be expected, as an external attribution would be predicted. This demonstrates the extent to which nurses take personal responsibility for their actions. However, those nurses where the outcome was more serious made a stronger internal attribution than those with the negligible outcome. Meurier *et al.* point out that all errors and near misses must be reported and acted upon as, although no harm occurred this time, next time there may be serious consequences. The behaviour of the nurses in the trivial outcome group suggests they would be more likely to ignore an error if the outcome were not serious. In terms of judging the quality of nursing care therefore, we have become too outcome driven and are possibly ignoring potentially dangerous errors if they do not produce a serious outcome *this time*. Next time it might be a different story.

This study does show nurses taking responsibility for their actions in such a way as to contradict a well-established area of social psychology. However, the study also opens up the possibility that nurses place too much emphasis on the outcome of care rather than the process involved. The jobs have been done and the patient discharged. These are things that can be counted and measured, therefore it is relatively easy to show that the instrumental dimension of care has been successfully completed. The psychosocial aspects of care are much more ongoing and concerned with the process of care. They are also difficult to measure with the result that they may become invisible and tend to be neglected, especially in busy areas.

Another aspect of care that has frequently given the author cause for concern is first aid. In teaching a wide range of post-registration students I am struck by the willingness with which they state that if they ever came across the scene of an accident they would cross over and walk on the other side of the road. This is the height of callous, uncaring behaviour and is usually justified on the grounds that they were told in their training to do this, they do not know anything about first aid and they are afraid of being sued. The flaws in this legal argument are exposed in Chapter 5. Such statements ignore the fact that every citizen has a duty of care to another and that as far as the UKCC are concerned, nurses *always* have a duty of care to any person. Did off duty nurses and other emergency workers in Omagh walk on by that dreadful day in August 1998 when a terrorist bomb caused such carnage? If any nurse has a moment's hesitation in deciding what to do at the scene of an accident, reflect upon what our colleagues in Northern Ireland have been through.

One final perspective on whether the theory of care in use matches the espoused theory concerns how nurses utilize research and the very nature of that research. There are actually two problems here, the first of which concerns the fact that nurses often fail to implement research findings or effectively utilize evidence as a base for their practice. Much has been written about this problem and the cause most frequently cited for nursing's failure to base care upon research are that nurses:

❑ Do not understand the way research papers are written up and any statistical analysis that may be included
❑ Are too busy to implement change
❑ Lack the authority to implement change. Uncooperative management, doctors and other nurses frustrate and block innovation
❑ Find it difficult to access the evidence and turn it into workable solutions.

The second problem is even more fundamental as it concerns the nature of the subject being researched itself, i.e. caring. Savage (1995) observes that as care is such a subjective concept, it is very difficult to define objectively and therefore to measure. If something cannot readily be measured then it becomes much harder to research. Nurse researchers already face the major problem of inadequate resources (hence the plethora of small-scale studies referred to earlier) to which we now add the fact that nursing care is a very elusive and difficult concept to capture and hence research. It is not surprising that much research into nursing has looked at topics such as nurses' attitudes rather than what nurses actually do. This lack of clinically relevant research further weakens the case for evidence-based caring practice.

Nursing therefore suffers from major difficulties in assembling an evidence base for caring practice and, even when such evidence is available, there are a range of barriers interfering with implementation. Although there is a wealth of literature passionately arguing what nursing care should consist of, the reality still frequently falls short of that rhetoric. One explanation is that the theory in use by many nurses, acquired over a substantial period of time, does not match the espoused theory of nurse academics and our professional bodies. I have suggested that the difficulties facing nursing research constitute a further reason why this should be, but it is not as simple as that. In order to gain further insights into why there is this mismatch between rhetoric and reality, it is necessary to look at the organization within which care takes place and this will be the purpose of the next chapter.

References

Argyris, C. and Schon, D. (1974). *Theory in Practice*. San Fransisco: Jossey Bass.

Baillie, L. (1996). A phenomenological study of the nature of empathy. *Journal of Advanced Nursing*, **24**, 1300–1308.

Benner, P. (1984). *From Novice to Expert*. Menlo Pk: Addison Wesley

Benner, P. and Wrubel, J. (1989). *The Primacy of Caring*. Menlo Pk: Addison Wesley

Byrne, G. and Heyman, R. (1997). Understanding nurses' communication with patients in A&E departments using a symbolic interactionist perspective. *Journal of Advanced Nursing*, **26**, 93–100.

Carveth, J. (1995). Perceived patient deviance and avoidance by nurses. *Nursing Research*, **44**, 173–178.

Cash, K. (1995). Benner and expertise in nursing: a critique. *International Journal of Nursing Studies*, **32**, 6, 527–534.

Cohen, J. and Stewart, I. (1994). *The Collapse of Chaos*. London: Penguin.

Dahlberg, K. (1996). Intersubjective meaning in holistic care: a Swedish perspective. *Nursing Science Quarterly*, **9**, 4, 147–151.

Dawkins, R. (1995). *River out of Eden*. London: Phoenix.

Darbyshire, P. (1994). Skilled expert practice, is it all in the mind? *Journal of Advanced Nursing*, **19**, 755–761.

English, I. (1993). Intuition as a function of the expert nurse; a critique of Benner's Novice to Expert Model. *Journal of Advanced Nursing*, **18**, 387–393.

Fletcher, J. (1997). Do nurses really care? Some unwelcome findings from recent research and inquiry. *Journal of Nursing Management*, **5**, 43–50.

Griffin, A. (1993). Holism in nursing; its meaning and value. *British Journal of Nursing*, **2**, 6, 310–312.

Handy, C. (1995). *The Gods of Management*. London: Arrow.

Hayter, M. (1996). Is non-judgemental care possible in the context of nurses' attitudes to patients' sexuality? *Journal of Advanced Nursing*, **24**, 662–666.

Henson, R. (1997). Analysis of the concept of mutuality. *Image; Journal of Nursing Scholarship*, **29**, 1, 77–81.

Homans, C. (1961). *Social Behaviour in its Elementary Forms*. New York: Harcourt Brace.

Jenny, J. and Logan, J. (1996). Caring and comfort metaphors used by patients in critical care. *Image: Journal of Nursing Scholarship*, **28**, 4, 349–352.

Lauri, S., Lepisto, M. and Kappeli, S. (1997). Patients' needs in hospital; nurses' and patients' views. *Journal of Advanced Nursing*, **25**, 339–346.

Leininger, M. (1977). *Caring, the essence and essential focus of nursing*. American Nurses Foundation (Nursing Research Report 14).

Leininger, M. (1981). *Caring; an Essential Human Need*. Thorofare, NJ: Charles B Slack.

MacDougal, G. (1997). Caring – a masculine perspective. *Journal of Advanced Nursing*, **25**, 809–813.

McKenna, G. (1993). Caring is the essence of nursing. *British Journal of Nursing*, **2**, 1, 72–75.

Meurier, C., Vincent, C. and Parmar, D. (1998). Nurses responses to severity dependent errors: a study of the causal attributions made by nurses following an error. *Journal of Advanced Nursing*, **27**, 349–354.

Montgomery, C. (1992). The spiritual connection: Nurses perception of the experience of caring. In: Gaut, D. (ed) *The Presence of Caring in Nursing*. New York: National League for Nursing.

Morrison, P. and Burnard, P. (1997). *Caring and Communicating* (2nd edn), London: Macmillan.

Morse, J., Solberg, M., Neander, W., Bottorff, J. and Johnson, J. (1990). Concepts of caring and caring as a concept. *Advances in Nursing Science*, **13**, 1–14.

Olson, D. (1997). When the patient causes the problem: the effect of patient responsibility on the nurse-patient relationship. *Journal of Advanced Nursing*, **26**, 515–522.

Olson, J. (1995). Relationships between nurse-expressed empathy and patient perceived empathy and patient distress. *Image: Journal of Nursing Scholarship*, **27**, 4, 317–321.

Olson, J. and Hanchett, E. (1997). Nurse-expressed empathy, patient outcomes and development of a middle range theory. *Image; Journal of Nursing Scholarship*, **29**, 1, 71–79.

Ovretveit, J. (1992). *Health Service Quality*. Oxford: Blackwell.

Pylkkannen, P. (1989). *The Search for Meaning; the New Spirit in Science and Philosophy*. Helsingfors: Crucible.

Price, V. and Archbold, J. (1997). What's it all about, empathy? *Nurse Education Today*, **17**, 106–111.

Raine, K. (1943). Parting. In: Heaney, S. and Hughes, T. (1997). *The School Bag*, London: Faber and Faber.

Rogers, C. (1957). The necessary and sufficient conditions of therapeutic personality change. *Journal of Consulting Psychology*, **21**, 95–103.

Sadler, J. (1997). Defining professional nurse caring; a triangulation study. *International Journal Human Caring*, **1**, 3, 12–21.

Savage, J. (1995). *Nursing Intimacy*. London: Scutari.

Stockwell, B. (1972). *The Unpopular Patient*. London: RCN.

Tuck, I., Harris, L., Renfro, T. and Lexvold, L. (1998). Care: A value expressed in philosophies of nursing services. *Journal of Professional Nursing*, **14**, 92–96.

Walsh, M. (1993). Pain and anxiety in A&E attenders. *Nursing Standard*, **7**, 26, 40–42.

Walsh, M. (1997a). *Models and Critical Pathways in Clinical Nursing*. London: Bailliere Tindall.

Walsh, M. (1997b). Accountability and intuition; justifying nursing practice. *Nursing Standard*, **11**, 23, 39–41.

Watson, J. (1997). The theory of human caring: retrospective and prospective. *Nursing Science Quarterly*, **10**, 1, 49–52.

Watson, R. and Lea, A. (1997). The caring dimensions inventory (CDI) Content validity, reliability and scaling. *Journal of Advanced Nursing*, **25**, 87–94.

White, S. (1997). Empathy; a literature review. *Journal of Clinical Nursing*, **6**, 253–257.

Wilde, M. (1997). The caring connection in nursing; a concept analysis. *International Journal of Human Caring*, **1**, 1, 18–24.

Yura, H. and Walsh, M. (1976). *Human Needs and the Nursing Process*. New York: Appleton Century Crofts.

CHAPTER 2

The organization
of care

'Twas brillig, and the slithy toves
Did gyre and gimble in the wabe:
All mimsy were the borogoves,
And the mome raths outgrabe.

Jabberwocky: Lewis Carroll (1872)

There are times when understanding the organization of anything in the NHS can seem as difficult as understanding Lewis Carroll's poem about the Jabberwocky. That is until you realize he has made it all up and it is complete nonsense! Perhaps there are times, as we saw in Chapter 1, that we can theorize about care to such an extent that what we have is a contender for Jabberwocky II, The Sequel, rather than a clear statement that is readily understood. Attempts at understanding organizations can also end up in a state of total 'jabberwocky', particularly when management jargon begins to creep in. This chapter will therefore try to offer some models that will help you break down the complexity of organizations into manageable pieces. However, as we have already seen, putting the pieces back together again is equally important if we are to avoid the errors of reductionism. The development of nursing practice will be reviewed in later chapters with one eye firmly on what happens when the pieces are put back together.

Care is not an abstract concept; it can only be understood in its context. It is therefore essential to look at the organization of caring activity if we are to see how the rhetoric of care translates into reality. Care is organized on several different levels starting with the one to one, nurse and patient relationship. Professional care does not happen spontaneously, it has to be planned and organized even when only a single nurse and patient are involved. However, in practice, nurses usually work with teams of other nurses and any one nurse will also have a group of patients for whom he or she is responsible. Organization therefore works at ward, department, treatment room or case load level. But there are more than nurses in the NHS, so we have to consider how the organization brings together all the other staff such as doctors, therapists, social workers and ancillary workers into Primary Care Teams, health centres, hospitals and NHS Trusts. But then these units need organizing together at regional and national level under the auspices of organizations such as the NHS Executive, the Scottish Office and the Department of Health, while the various national bodies that regulate the health professions have their own national perspective. The nurse therefore operates within a complex series of organizations, each of which will have its own history, traditions and, therefore, culture. By analogy it is rather like a series of Russian dolls, one nesting within the other.

If we go back and start at the beginning, we are looking at the individual nurse and how he or she might organize care with his or her colleagues. Broadly speaking there have been four approaches starting with the task-focused system that was dominant until well into the 1970s. Patients were broken up into tasks and each nurse assigned specific tasks for that shift with the result that it was very difficult for a nurse to get to know a patient as a whole person. This was followed by patient allocation which saw one, two or more nurses given a group of patients to care for during a shift, but come the next shift they would have another group of patients, preventing any real close nurse–patient relationships from developing. Team nursing allowed a group of nurses to care for the same patients all the time and, as a result, nurses and patients started to get to know each other and continuity of care became established as well as a sense of teamworking. The final stage in this evolutionary process was the introduction of primary nursing which gave experienced nurses 24-hour responsibility for a group of patients, while associate nurses provided care in the primary nurses' absence. Each of these systems makes different basic assumptions about patients and the nature of nursing care, which are presented in simplified form below. They can be seen as a spectrum of care with the patient progressively having more opportunity to become an active partner in care, while the nurse sees the patient increasingly as a person. There is also a progressive increase in the accountability of the individual nurse. The issues of accountability and responsibility will be explored in detail in Chapter 6.

❑ Task: Patient is a passive recipient of tasks performed for him/her.

Nursing is concerned with getting the jobs done. There is no need to know the patient as a person, in fact it is probably better not to get involved at all. Responsibility for patients (and knowledge about care) rests with nurse in charge.

❑ Patient allocation: Patient is seen as someone to pass on to another group of nurses at the end of the shift.

Nursing is still concerned with getting the jobs done but at least the patient starts to become a whole person. It is still difficult to appreciate the role of psychosocial factors in health. Responsibility for care rests with a group leader for single shift.

❑ Team nursing: Patient can now be seen as a whole person who can be a partner in their care as there is time to get to know him/her.

Nursing can now provide continuity of care. This means that the nurse can now focus on the psychosocial dimensions of care as well as the physical. Nurse–patient relationship building is facilitated. Teamwork becomes very important however, as team members have to trust each other and share long-term responsibility for care in an accountable fashion.

❏ Primary nursing: Patient seen as an individual person who is a partner in care, assuming they are willing to be so.

Nursing has strong similarities with team nursing but with a stronger element of individual accountability. Associate nurses are responsible and accountable to primary nurses while primary nurses carry 24 hours per day accountability for their patients.

A key question to ask about the organization of care is, for whose benefit is it being organized? There are several players each with different perspectives and priorities of their own. These include the patient, the nurses giving care, the nurse in charge carrying overall accountability (e.g. ward Sister, District Nursing Sister), doctors and other professional staff (PAMS) such as physiotherapists and social workers. The reader might reflect upon these four different systems of organizing care and rank the five key players listed above in order of who stands to benefit most in each of the four systems. Table 2.1 sets up the different players, try to fill it in based upon your experience.

Take each system in turn, ranking the key players so that the one who benefits most is 1 and the one who benefits least is 5.

Table 2.1 Who Benefits Most from the Organization of Care?

System	Key players				
	Patient	*Doctor*	*Nurse*	*Nurse in charge*	*Other*
PAMS					
Task oriented care					
Patient allocation					
Team nursing					
Primary nursing					

Having completed Table 2.1, rank the five players in general order of power – 1 is the most powerful and 5 the least powerful. Experience of working this exercise with students produces some intense debate, but there is usually a general consensus that primary nursing stands to benefit the patient most, while task-centred nursing benefits the nurse in charge most and also is the best fit for the medical model. When power is considered, the doctor and ward sister are generally ranked as the two most powerful players with the patient the least powerful. This mismatch explains a lot of the difficulty in implementing primary nursing and, in general, moving nursing care towards the ideal of patients as partners in care.

Whether it is the way care is organized by individual or groups of nurses or the way those nurses fit into a series of bigger organizations, one of the major factors in understanding the delivery of care is the organizational context within which it occurs. In order to further this analysis, it is therefore useful to look at the thinking of some American and British organizational gurus in order to grasp better the connection between organization and care. The analytical tools of Peters and Waterman (McKinseys 7S Analysis) together with the thinking of Charles Handy will therefore be applied to the organization of care.

The McKinsey 7S analysis and the climate of care

The work of Peters and Waterman (1982) led them to draw up an analytical framework for investigating organizations and how they work. They discovered seven key areas, which conveniently all begin with the letter 'S'. Charles Handy's contribution is to look at organizational culture. There are two significant points to be made by combining these areas of work.

❑ The organization has to be internally consistent otherwise discontinuities will generate friction and disagreement leading to a dysfunctional organization. The 7S analysis allows a thorough examination to be made to see if the organization is internally consistent with its culture and values.
❑ The culture of the organization has to be the right one for the business in hand, i.e. it has to be fit for purpose.

As you read through the rest of this chapter, reflect upon your own clinical area using the 7S framework. It will help you to understand better what is happening and as a result gain insights which will facilitate the development of care.

Shared values

Values are the things that matter to someone. If an organization is to work they should be shared by all members of staff, hence the writing of mission statements and philosophies of care. Unfortunately, mission statements are usually long winded, pious statements that nobody can remember and which consequently are of little practical use. A good mission statement should reflect the one thing that matters most to all concerned and be written in tabloid newspaper headlines. Whatever the reader may think of the content of the tabloid press, they do have the knack of writing pithy headlines that catch the eye and stick in the memory.

If different members of the nursing team value different things, it is going to be difficult to get everybody working together. If care is the main value, then it is important that all staff mean the same thing by care. As we have seen, care means different things to different people and, in nursing, it has traditionally meant getting the jobs done without any emotional involvement or feeling. It is only recently that the value of empathy has been recognized and it is starting to become permissible to experience emotions as a nurse. If care is at the core of your mission statement, check that both the older and younger members of the team have the same understanding of what care means. You should also consider the extent to which other professional groups share the same values as nurses and at least recognize your differences. However, the more we talk of multidisciplinary teams, the more important it becomes to share values within the team rather than have a dominant value system that suborns others. Can the objective values of biomedical science be reconciled with the more subjective values of a social science such as nursing? If not, then staff should at least recognize their differences and respect where they are each coming from rather than have one value system imposed on the rest.

Structure and culture

The culture of an organization reflects the commonly held beliefs, values and attitudes of its members. It usually owes a lot to history and is learnt by new recruits as part of their socialization process. It is also remarkably stable and acts as a barrier to change within any organization be it the NHS, nursing in general, or your particular health centre or ward. The all-pervasive and often unconscious nature of culture means that it determines a great deal of the structures that exist in any care environment and consequently the way in which the care itself is delivered.

A very perceptive analysis of organizational culture has been provided by Charles Handy (1995), who describes four main types and, rather whimsically, names each one after an appropriate Greek god. They may be summarized as follows:

Apollo: The role culture. It is characterized by order and routine for Apollo was the Greek god of order. There is a strong hierarchy and the work a person does depends upon their carefully defined role, rules, routines and position in the hierarchy. Such an organization is very stable and rule bound; it only works well when tomorrow is like yesterday.

Dominant values are logic, reason, routines and procedures. The structure can be visualized as a series of ladders side by side with each ladder representing a professional group. Staff work their way up their own professional hierarchy step by step, but there are wide gaps between the ladders hence there are major communication problems between groups of staff.

Zeus: The power culture. This sort of organization is dominated by a single powerful individual who can be conceptualized as being the spider at the centre of the web. He or she is the only person who knows the full picture. This kind of organization can react to situations very quickly as Zeus tends to tell people what to do directly rather than rely upon consultation, discussion or written reports. Staff also tend to do things according to how Zeus would wish them done without needing to be told, as they have learnt there is only one way of doing things and that is the way of Zeus, the King of the Gods, sitting on Mount Olympus! Dominant values are power, personality and risk taking. The structure can be seen as a spider's web with the dominant person sitting at the centre. He or she is the only one who has the full picture.

Athenae: The task culture. A different approach here. This is all about teamwork and involves teams of staff working on specific problems with a large degree of autonomy. Success is judged in terms of outcomes and problems solved. Power is derived from knowledge rather than hierarchy or force of personality as in the previous two examples. Dominant values are group work, democracy, achieving results and output. The structure is rather like a net or matrix in that there are self-contained groups of people spaced around the organization, but no sense of hierarchy.

Dionysus: The individualistic or existentialist culture. Dionysus was the god of song and wine and presumably chosen by Handy for his hedonistic, self-indulgent nature. In this culture you tend to find strong individualists with no apparent organizational structure other than a loose agglomeration of individuals who combine together from time to time, when it suits them to do so, for some specific purpose. Individuals are often well educated and expert in their fields. The dominant values are independence, individuality and personal expertise. The structure can best be described as unstructured, a loose agglomeration of individuals with no sense of hierarchy.

The nurse will recognize examples of each of these different cultural types in the NHS. Nursing with its hierarchies and clinical grading is a good example of an Apollo role culture, while the traditional ward sister running a largely task-oriented ward is an example of a latterday Zeus. Some individual doctors behave like Zeus but Dionysus is often a better description of the culture of medicine. Team nursing can resemble Athenae, as might a well-run primary health care team, while Dionysus is a good description of many GP practices and medical directorates within acute hospitals. Dionysus could also be seen as describing a well-developed primary nursing system.

A moment's reflection will reveal that the different cultures and structures have a profound effect upon the delivery of care, particularly if you try to locate the patient somewhere within the structure. The role culture of Apollo has several serious weaknesses, not least of which is that it is not able to cope with the rapidly changing world of health care we are now in. Tomorrow is not going to be the same as yesterday. As the boundaries between nursing and medicine dissolve, shift and change so do nursing and medical roles, thus we need a more flexible change-oriented culture with structures that facilitate change. A further weakness of the hierarchical structure is that it leaves the patient at the bottom of the hierarchy, the lowest rung on the ladder, furthest away from the nurse with the most expertise. The role of the patient is also changing so a culture that is wedded to the traditional passive patient role is no longer fit for purpose. The row of ladders structure (one ladder for the nursing team, one for the medical team etc.) also has the problem that communication tends to be a one way process. Messages are handed down each ladder, one rung at a time, but little comes back up while there is no cross communication at all between ladders.

The main problem with the Zeus structure is that the only person who has the whole picture is Zeus! Other staff trying to care for the patient only see part of the picture which renders holistic care impossible, makes for misunderstandings ('I thought you were doing that' or ' we've done that already') and low job satisfaction. There is no room for the patient in this spider's web, therefore the patient is again a passive recipient of care. The ability of the Zeus structure to perform very quickly and its ability to feed off adrenalin, however, means that there are certain emergency areas where such a structure is wholly appropriate such as in the field of resuscitation (A&E trauma team or the hospital arrest team).

Athenae has the chance to offer more positive working relationships that incorporate the patient into the team. The notion of patient as partner in care can be realized in such a team structure. The problem is whether the dominant NHS cultures of Zeus and Apollo will permit Athenae the autonomy and resources to flourish. There is also the problem that a strong personality may take over the team and reduce it to a power culture (Zeus). This is a particular difficulty in primary care teams where the assumption is often that the doctor will always be team captain. Athenae requires expertise and staff to be accountable, knowledgeable practitioners. Evidence-based practice should underpin this approach.

The primary nursing system of care could look like Dionysus. Clinical nurse specialists within a trust or nurse practitioners might also be thought of in the same way. It offers freedom from hierarchy, a fair degree of autonomy and facilitates patient involvement in care. Nurses, however, have to have a high degree of expertise and the confidence to operate in this style. Clinical supervision, peer review or some other support network is essential to ensure support in what could be an isolated style of working. Individualistic cultures require effective clinical audit to give the feedback on performance that might otherwise be obtained from peers within a team culture (Athenae).

Staff

Identifying the staff who work in a care environment is a worthwhile exercise. You may find there are various people who you never thought of as having anything to do with care such as the ward cleaner or practice receptionist who may spend more time talking with patients than the registered nurse. Staff such as these make a vital contribution which may be unrecognized. Making their contribution visible is likely to make care more effective and help generate a better team atmosphere, which is particularly important if staff are trying to develop a culture of teamwork (Athenae). What is crucial is to think through the value systems of all the staff involved and see if they match the values of the organization. In recent years we have seen an obvious mismatch in the NHS with the values of the market place being imposed upon clinicians by managers. Peters and Waterman (1982) predict that a major unconformity in value systems will lead to failure. The notion of clinical governance offers an opportunity for all health professionals to re-establish caring values as the common value system in health care.

Style

The management or leadership style of those in senior positions is crucial to the functioning of the organization. Within a role culture, the management style is likely to be rational with an insistence upon rules, procedures and protocol. This approach does not allow for flexibility, creativity, experimentation and new ideas, the very things that we need most in the rapidly changing environment of care that nurses work in today. If we believe that patient need should drive health care then that should be the starting point for developing responsive services. Unfortunately, a rational manager in a role culture that values order above all else will tend to start by thinking in terms of the status quo; what staff are available? what do these staff do (roles)? what do the regulations permit? what do we usually do? This bureaucratic mind set will fail to meet the need for new services because it will try to answer new problems with old solutions and usually conclude that nothing can be done because the rules will not allow it. Nurse practitioners have sometimes fallen foul of this obsession with traditional roles and boundaries (not least the UKCC) but, where staff have worked on problems unencumbered by traditional roles and hierarchies, creative and workable solutions have been found.

The Zeus culture lends itself to what is known as a transforming style of management which is about getting others to do things by whatever means possible. The views of the individual nurse do not matter as long as he or she does as he or she is told. This is the authoritarian legacy of the so-called good old days and is congruent with the patriarchal, doctor knows best style of patient management which also exists in the parallel, matriarchal universe, of nurse knows best. If we wish to be consistent in our approach to care and move patients away from being the passive recipients of instructions and medications (which they usually ignore when they go home), then we, as nurses and doctors, must move away from the same style of management in our daily work.

The task and individualistic cultures of Athenae and Dionysus respectively require very different management and leadership styles. A team approach requires a more humanistic style that involves respect, democracy and valuing other members of the team. It is obvious how this style connects with the kind of values we wish to promote in developing patients as partners in care. The nurse who respects the patient's views and wishes and who is prepared to negotiate over care is likely to achieve a higher degree of cooperation with treatment than Zeus with all his thunderbolts. Dionysus requires empowerment, for this is a loose unstructured collection of talented individuals. Leadership of such a group requires the empowerment of the individuals towards a common goal (shared values again). The nurse working in such an environment should find empowering the patient, or another member of staff such as an associate nurse to be normal practice. There are some patients, however, who may prefer the nurse or doctor to play at Zeus, absolving them of the need to think about and take responsibility for their care. Comments such as, 'Just do what you think is best doctor', or, 'I'll leave it up to you nurse', may still be heard fairly frequently.

A crucial point about management style is that whenever a new manager is appointed, their style has to fit the culture of the organization otherwise the ensuing mismatch will be dysfunctional. A group of staff who have become used to working as a team with a high degree of autonomy and collective responsibility for decisions will not take kindly to having a manager imposed upon them who wishes to control everything. The reverse is equally true. Deliberately putting a new person in charge as an attempt to change the existing culture is unlikely to work unless accompanied by a range of other steps in support of change. This is well illustrated by the work of Binnie and Titchen (1993) as their action research project set about changing the culture of a traditional largely task-focused ward to primary nursing. Their paper could have been titled from Zeus to Dionysus (via Athenae) as that was the journey they undertook!

Systems and procedures

Reflection upon the various systems that nurses have used in order to carry out patient care shows that they can be fitted into the various cultures that Handy has described. The point that Peters and Waterman (1982) make is that the organization of care will only work if the approach is consistent across all 7 Ss and if it is the right approach.

The traditional task allocation approach to nursing belongs within the role culture of Apollo. The patient was broken up into a series of tasks of varying complexity (and prestige) and different nurses performed those tasks as appropriate to their position in the hierarchy. The procedure manual and Sister's opinions governed the practice of nursing while a series of books recorded baths, bowel movements and dressing changes.

The introduction of the nursing process had the beneficial effect of doing away with all the different books as patients were now supposed to be assessed as people, their care planned and written out in a single coherent document. Unfortunately the task-oriented culture of nursing was so ingrained that, although the paperwork changed, it was a long time before anything else did and care still remained task focused for many years.

Attempts at change led to the notion of allocating a group of patients typically to one or two nurses to care for during a shift. This patient allocation system at least allowed the nurse to be responsible for all the care received by a patient during a shift but, as the allocations changed from shift to shift and day to day, nurses did not really get to know their patients and continuity of care was lacking. If the ward sister was a powerful character then a Zeus culture could continue as it might have done under the old task allocation system, otherwise the Apollonian culture would prevail. True teamworking or individual accountability for care could not flourish under this system as it required a different culture.

Team nursing or the operation of a truly multidisciplinary primary care team, requires the team-based culture of Athenae. In this system, individuals work together as a team with a high degree of autonomy and are judged by their results. The team therefore operates democratically and shares decisions. Dividing a ward into two teams, allocating patients to each and letting the staff get on with their nursing care, requires the ward sister to abandon the role of Zeus, she has to trust her staff and not be continually checking up on them. Clinical audit and good documentation of care are essential. This allows the sister to be monitoring performance discreetly and is consistent with team culture in that results are what matter. The weaknesses and problems associated with the nursing process are therefore going to cause problems with such an approach, as the good quality documentation that is needed may not be available. Critical pathways with their sharp focus upon outcomes offer a more promising alternative to the nursing process. The sister who insists upon enforcing procedures upon the teams and who cannot resist the temptation to interfere with their work will render team nursing ineffectual. The re-establishment of hierarchies within teams will also undermine the operation of such a system as they contradict the cultural norms of teamwork. One valuable offshoot of a democratic teamworking culture is that it makes it natural to have the patient as an equal member of the team, involved in all decisions about care.

The individualistic culture of Dionysus is consistent with primary nursing. The primary nurses work together in a loose association but each must accept total accountability for the care given to their patients due to the individualistic nature of the system. In team nursing decisions can be shared, but here the primary nurse carries the sole responsibility and therefore the ultimate accountability. Webb and Pontin (1996) report that this has mixed effects in terms of stress as, while greater responsibility can increase stress, it can also reduce it by giving nurses more control over their work. All registered nurses are of course accountable to the UKCC, to their employers and to their patients. It would be counterproductive if primary nurses were to take this accountability issue too literally and as a result not consult with their colleagues about decisions. The most important person of all when it comes to consultation, however, is the patient and primary nursing offers the best opportunity for such real partnerships in care to develop.

Good documentation is essential for, if the primary nurse takes the individualistic nature of this culture to extremes, nobody else knows what is supposed to be happening! Webb and Pontin (1996) discovered a substantial increase in both the volume and types of communication subsequent upon the introduction of primary nursing in the wards they investigated, yet one ward coordinator still felt vulnerable to negligence claims as she felt did not know what was going on. There is, therefore, within such an individualistic culture a greater than ever need for effective communication. This suggests there is a powerful argument for the use of shared, multidisciplinary documentation, such as critical pathways, rather than the increasingly discredited, traditional nursing process (Wilson, 1997). The primary nurse is the ideal person to manage a critical pathway as he or she has the broad overview of the whole patient that is so essential. The primary nurse must also be directly involved in care, not just a manager of care (Meade, 1991). It is also usual to provide the patient with their own copy of the critical pathway which enhances the patient as partner in care concept.

Nurse practitioners are developing a whole range of new roles and they, too, often fit into this individualistic culture almost by default, as they tend to be relatively rare and potentially quite isolated. The attitude of other nurses towards nurse practitioners is equally important in determining whether they evolve in a predominantly individualistic culture or become more integrated into health care teams.

Strategies

The term strategies, in this context, refers to how you do things and the processes used to make things happen. Care took place within a role culture by virtue of routine and ritual, the procedure manual ruled care and individual nurses were absolved from the responsibility of thinking for themselves. The hierarchical nature of such a culture ensured that it was seen as natural to split tasks into a hierarchy of importance which governed which grades of staff did what. Sister traditionally did the ward round, staff nurses did drug rounds and dressings while 'other ranks' (students and the nursing auxiliaries) did everything else. Nurses were used to routinized, ritualistic care. When the nursing process came along, however, they had to assess patient needs and plan care on an individual basis, in other words, think for themselves. Not surprisingly, they found this difficult and many nursing process care plans were routinized and lacking in any individuality or relationship to the assessment which should have informed them. Davis *et al.* (1994), in their investigation of nursing process documentation, showed how nurses struggled with just these problems, revealing poor documenta- tion of assessment and little if any individualized care planning that could be related to the assessment, especially in the psychosocial domain. Traditional nurse training reinforced these behaviours as it discouraged independent thinking while, historically, the whole culture of nursing was rooted in the Victorian traditions of obedience and subservience.

A power culture needs such obedience of course and it is therefore not surprising that a common strategy for getting things done in health care has simply been telling somebody else to do it. Directives, unaccompanied by explanations or justifications were the traditional way of getting things done in nursing. Many doctors today still expect nurses to obey their instructions without question and are very nonplussed when nurses query, challenge or offer alternative suggestions. Following orders was not an acceptable defence at the Nuremburg war criminal trials at the end of the Second World War and it is not an acceptable defence today, whether the nurse is being called to account by the UKCC or in a court of law.

The power culture of Zeus is therefore still apparent and is often rationalized as clinical judgement. The phrase 'in my clinical judgement' was once all powerful and stemmed any dissent in the ranks. However, the growth of the evidence-based practice movement has now effectively challenged this position which was often a smokescreen anyway. Nurses should beware falling into the trap explaining practice by such phrases as 'clinical judgement' or, alternatively, 'I was only doing what I was told', as evidence to justify practice is essential if the nurse really is going to be an accountable practitioner. Primary nurses must expect associate nurses and students to question their plans of care from time to time and be professionally mature enough to justify their care through recourse to evidence rather than falling back on 'clinical judgement' alone or deploying a Benner-like 'expert/intuitive practice' argument. The legal implications of being unable to offer evidence in support of practice will be explored later (Chapter 5).

The team culture requires different strategies for getting things done as simply telling people to do things is at odds with a collective sense of collegiality and the notion that each member of the team has a valued contribution to make. Alternatively, recourse to routine and ritual stifle the living daylights out of the creative thinking necessary for a team approach to problem solving. The team is typically faced with planning and carrying out care for a group of patients. The team product is that care and the job they have to do boils down to problem solving. The strategies required are therefore flexible thinking, research (trial and error is a simple form of research), asking others for advice and looking at the evidence. These strategies all facilitate the main task of problem solving.

The individualistic culture that underpins primary nursing logically requires the practitioner to rely upon individual judgement. If that individual judgement is based on evidence gathered from a range of sources such as research and the literature, patient preferences, discussion with colleagues and personal experience derived from critical reflection upon practice, the nurse will be more likely to make the right decisions. However, if personal prejudices and outdated practices influence judgement, the patient will be poorly served. Evidence-based practice is therefore a strategy that is essential if effective care is to be based within either a team or individualistic culture.

Skills

The skills which staff possess and the way they are acquired will also vary according to the culture of the organization providing care. Within a role culture, skills are clearly linked to job descriptions and grades. To a large extent skills are prescribed by the job description and paper qualifications are required as proof of competency before a person is hired. The whole sorry saga of clinical grading reflects the kind of morass this can lead into. Nurse practitioners are another example of how this culture does nursing no favours. They are challenging the established order in a most fundamental way. Unfortunately, by seeking to add medical skills to their therapeutic tool kit they have become labelled by some as mini-doctors. This mistake stems from thinking in terms of specific roles requiring specific skills and then reversing that thought process so that if a person has certain skills they must have a certain role. I have some gardening skills but that does not make me Alan Titchmarsh, while my ability to kick a football does not make me Alan Shearer! The nurse practitioner has acquired some extra medical skills to help him or her fulfil *a new role, not an existing medical role.*

The power culture of Zeus has a different approach to skills. There are no tightly defined roles and logically determined skills, rather the transforming style of management means that staff do anything the boss can get them to do. Skills are acquired on an *ad hoc* basis without too much concern about national guidelines and statutory bodies. If a member of staff cannot do something they have to find out how, and quickly. The approach is that of a 'can do attitude' which means that, in certain circumstances, things can happen very quickly. In health care, however, there must be concerns about the safety of what is being done. The old medical adage of 'see one, do one, teach one' fits into this culture very neatly and it illuminates some of the worrying ways that nurses have expanded their practice in recent years without adequate preparation.

This again raises the issue of the failure of the UKCC to deal with nurse practitioner development. The lack of any national recognition of the title means there are no national standards defining the role and hence the education needed to practise safely. Many nurses have suddenly found their role expanding on the basis of a short, *ad hoc*, medical training programme, resulting in the title of nurse practitioner. Their role expansion has usually been in response to urgent service need brought about by medical staffing problems. When the nurse practitioner role is carefully thought out and based upon a nurse led education programme at first degree level, as the RCN recommend, the result is likely to be beneficial to all concerned. When expansion takes place as a quick fix within a medically dominated, Zeus-like 'can do' culture however, there have to be serious concerns about the safety of the end product and the well being of the staff involved (Crouch, 1996). This is no way to develop nursing practice.

Where teamwork is the pervading culture and output is what is prized most (care in the case of nursing), skills and education tend to be highly valued. Courses are therefore seen as the main route to the acquisition of skills. Skills of course involve more than mechanical dexterity as the person must understand the rationale behind any skill. Good communication and the ability to build interpersonal relationships are skills fundamental to any teamworking. These are skills which did not feature too highly in the nurse training of yore and which have been a very welcome addition to recent nursing education. Our medical colleagues have often not had the benefit of such training however, and, at times, it shows. True teamworking involving doctors does need to address this issue.

In a more individualistic culture, skill acquisition is often left up to the individual to pursue. However, it is essential that staff are well educated and have the necessary confidence in their skills to operate in such an individualistic way as there are fewer institutional safety nets. This mode of operation is one with which few nurses are familiar and it does require self-confidence, allied with the ability to manage risk and uncertainty. Isolation can lead to a failure to recognize when things are not going well or to the individual falling behind the times. Critical reflection upon practice and networking skills are essential, together with the skills of accessing up-to-date evidence in order that practice be kept in line with current thinking and guidelines.

Summary

This chapter demonstrates that the organization of nursing care was characterized by a fragmented and task-oriented approach which involved the minimum communication with the patient and which was deliberately designed to prevent the nurse really getting to know the patient. The more recent approaches such as team and primary nursing offer the nurse the opportunity to build meaningful relationships with the patient who, in turn, may become much more actively involved in his or her care. This progress is consistent with much of the literature about care discussed in Chapter 1, however, as we also saw in Chapter 1, the practice of care often falls short of the rhetoric. The issues of culture and organization discussed in this chapter offer at least part of the explanation as to why this should be. The reader is encouraged to analyse their own place of work using the McKinsey 7S Framework and also to reflect upon the ideas of Charles Handy about organizational culture. Blaming the theory–practice gap upon lack of staff and out of touch nurse tutors will not resolve the problem. While staffing is an issue which cannot be ignored and there may well be a small number of nurse tutors who are out of touch with clinical practice, there are some fundamental problems nearer home in the clinical area which have to be faced up to and recognized. The culture and organization of care may well be the major barriers standing between the ideals of nursing and its reality in practice.

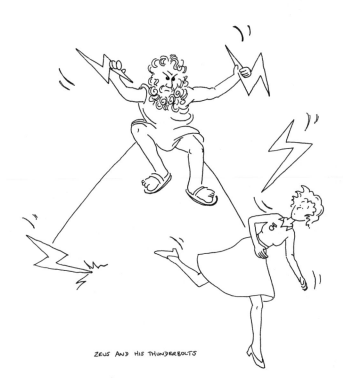

ZEUS AND HIS THUNDERBOLTS

References

Binnie, A. and Titchen, A. (1993). What am I meant to be doing? Putting theory into practice and back again with the new nursing roles. *Journal of Advanced Nursing*, **18**, 1054–1065.

Carroll, L. (1872). Jabberwocky. In: Heaney, S. and Hughes, T. (1997). *The School Bag*. London: Faber and Faber.

Crouch, S. (1996). Professionals, myth or reality? *Nursing Management*, **3**, 6, 12–13.

Davis, B., Billings, J. and Ryland, R. (1994). Evaluation of the nursing process. *Journal of Advanced Nursing*, **19**, 960–968.

Handy, C. (1995). *The Gods of Management*. London: Arrow.

Meade, D. (1991). An evaluation tool for primary nursing. *Nursing Standard*, **6**, 1, 37–39.

Peters, T. and Waterman, R. (1982). *In Pursuit of Excellence*. London: Harper Row.

Webb, C. and Pontin, D. (1996). Introducing primary nursing; nurses' opinions. *Journal of Clinical Nursing*, **5**, 351–358.

Wilson, J. (1997). *Integrated Care Management; The Path to Success?* Oxford: Butterworth-Heinemann.

CHAPTER 3

Is nursing a profession?

'All professions are a conspiracy against the laity'

George Bernard Shaw (1907)

Introduction

Nursing has spent much time and effort over the last couple of decades trying to establish itself as a profession, without actually questioning what a profession is and, therefore, considering whether we should try to join this exclusive club. I readily admit to being a dedicated follower of 'professionalism' in the past but the 1990s has seen some serious questions asked about professionalism which are neatly captured by George Bernard Shaw's famous dictum quoted above. The UKCC seems to have assumed that nursing is a profession already hence documents such as the *Scope of Professional Practice* and the *Code of Professional Conduct*. This assumption has to be questioned. Nursing needs to step back from the headlong pursuit of professional status and pause for some critical reflection concerning whether this is desirable or whether we might be better served pursuing a different agenda.

What makes a profession?

Ask this question to any group of nurses and you will quickly be able to fill a flip chart with answers. This approach to understanding profession-alism is sometimes called the trait model and assumes that there is a series of common characteristics that can be found in all professions. Typical answers given from post-registration students of my own include a knowledge base, a code of ethics, altruism (doing things for the benefit of others rather than self), commitment to public service, prestige, trustworthiness, selection, training and a qualification process.

Sociologists have studied professions in an attempt to draw up a list of traits or characteristics that can be used as a yardstick against which to measure any occupational group. Haralambos and Holborn (1995) have summarized this literature and consider that the following are the main attributes of a profession:

1 A systematic and organized knowledge base

2 Public service and altruism

3 Codes of ethics and regulation of professional conduct

4 High levels of reward.

Three of the four are contained in the list of attributes described above, however the fourth point clearly does not apply to nursing, any of the *professions* allied to medicine (PAMS) or several other occupations that might be regarded as attaining professional status such as teaching or social work. This is the first indication that this view of professionalism might be problematical. We will return to this point later.

The traits outlined above fit within a view that has been described by sociologists as the functionalist interpretation of professions. This account sees professions as having a special place in society and it is their unique role to help that society function effectively. Historically, professions have therefore acquired high prestige and an ideal of public service. Key areas in all societies include the law, medicine, the military and religion together with, in more advanced societies, the ability to design and build great buildings. Judges and lawyers, priests and doctors, generals and admirals have occupied these high status positions from the times of ancient Greece and Rome through to the present day.

The professions were concerned with the fundamentals of making a society work. Key central values such as law and order, security, health and religion are so important and the practitioner acquires such specialized and advanced levels of knowledge that the ordinary person ('client') has to submit to the authority of the professional. This automatic submission to professional authority led to the need for strict internal regulation and an ethical code of conduct by the professions in order to avoid exploitation and the acquisition of a bad reputation which would damage their status. The crucial importance of the work that profession-als do also explains the high levels of reward enjoyed by these people.

Nursing has based its claim for professional status upon this functionalist account of professions, listing a series of traits which reflect the altruistic attributes of a profession. This combination of trait and functionalist ideas results in a framework against which any occupational group, such as nursing, can measure its professionalism. The assumption has tended to be that either nursing was a profession already or was working towards the achievement of enough traits to become one.

A typical analysis of this argument is presented by Keogh (1997). He argues that nursing has the attributes of a profession and lists the following aspects of nursing which meet the classical definition given above:

Nursing:

❑ Has a body of specialized knowledge
❑ Uses the scientific method to enlarge that body of knowledge
❑ Education is now located within the university sector
❑ Has control over its professional policy and activity
❑ Is practised by nurses who have a lifetime commitment and
   dedication to nursing
❑ Offers a service to the public
❑ Has professional autonomy.

Consideration of these points reveals that there are serious flaws in this argument. Nursing is something of a magpie when it comes to a knowledge base as we have drawn heavily upon the biomedical and social sciences for our theoretical underpinning. There has been a substantial amount of effort in North America among nurse academics to generate a body of knowledge which is unique to nursing, much of it, however, remains incomprehensible due to the arcane language such authors use and has consequently attracted little support from the average nurse. Furthermore, to claim that expert nursing is intuitive as Benner does (1984) downgrades the role of scientific knowledge and evidence within nursing. Finally, there is the criticism of many authors that nursing practice is frequently based upon ritual, tradition, external authority and the *attitudes* and *beliefs* of nurses, rather than knowledge or hard evidence.

The use of the scientific method to enlarge nursing's knowledge base has run into serious difficulty as many writers have urged nursing to abandon quantitative research in favour of qualitative. By definition, qualitative data cannot be measured objectively, generalized or used to make predictions about future events, all of which are key components of the scientific method. Qualitative research lacks the elements of control and randomization which allow the researcher to link cause and effect. The issue of causality is fundamental to the scientific method. It translates into nursing when you can say research shows dressing X probably *causes* a wound to heal more rapidly than another can or that increased patient teaching probably *causes* a reduction in postoperative pain and complications. The academics who are urging nursing to follow a different path to the scientific method do nursing a disservice and also rather undermine the validity of Keogh's arguments.

The assertion that the transfer of nursing education into higher education confers the status of professionalism upon nursing has problems. While the other professions have long been at home in the university sector and are all graduate entry, nurses in the UK remain largely a non-graduate occupational group who seem to distrust degree level education. Many nurses are critical of academia, preferring a skills-based apprenticeship training to an academic education. Even the modest moves made in the Dip HE reforms known as Project 2000 have been the subject of much criticism which is grossly unfair to those students who have qualified from such programmes in the last few years. Fletcher (1997) has argued that nursing education must strive to develop a coherent body of knowledge based upon the research of those who teach if it is to make any progress towards becoming a profession with the same status as medicine or law. Sadly, the majority of those who teach do not have the time and/or inclination to become involved in such research and the dismal showing of nursing in the 1996 Research Assessment Exercise (RAE) when compared to other disciplines does not augur well for the future. Simply being in Higher Education does not make a profession if the culture of nursing remains hostile to research and academic development.

The issue of professional control and activity will be dealt with in more detail in Chapter 4. There has been a welcome increase in the amount of control nurses have over their professional policy and activity in the 1990s, but there are still major problems. Consider the sorry saga of prescribing rights for nurses and the growth of nurse practitioner roles as two examples. Despite being proposed in a Government Report (Cumberledge Report, 1988), 10 years on we have made little progress as successive governments have frustrated attempts to afford prescribing rights for nurses while the UKCC, despite being the regulatory body for nursing, has failed to engage the nurse practitioner movement and show real leadership. The power in health care still rests with the medical profession and increasingly with the new breed of managers who have emerged since the late 1980s. These two groups exert significant control over nursing and interfere with nursing's control of its own agenda. Various writers have looked at nursing both from a feminist perspective and also using a critical social theory framework to argue that nurses remain in many ways an oppressed group with little control over their occupation (Ford and Walsh, 1994). This view is at odds with Keogh's assertion about power and control.

While nursing clearly has a code of ethics, there is a problem with the assertion that nurses have a lifetime commitment. Increasing levels of staff turnover and the recruitment and retention crisis that is currently causing major problems to the NHS suggest that many nurses do not have a lifetime commitment as they fail to complete their basic nursing education or leave nursing never to return. There is a considerable debate about whether this is due to poor salary and conditions of service or a feeling of being overworked and undervalued by poor employers, perhaps both play a part in differing amounts for different nurses. Either way, the steady loss of nurses from the health care field is a serious threat to the long-term viability of the NHS.

The final attribute considered by Keogh is autonomy which, he admits, is difficult for nurses to achieve. The arguments for nursing's traditional subservience to medicine are well known and as long as this is the case, nursing will not be able to claim a large degree of autonomy. Crouch (1996) summarizes the evidence for nursing's subservience to medicine and is also critical of the changes made by the UKCC to the *Code of Professional Conduct* (UKCC, 1992) which now merely requires nurses to *report* unsatisfactory standards of care rather than *take action* as the Code originally did. Given the disempowered state of nursing it could be argued that the UKCC are only being realistic, but it certainly reflects the lack of autonomy nursing has if its regulatory body cannot bring itself to require direct action from nurses when they encounter unsatisfactory standards of care. In Crouch's view, therefore, nursing lacks the autonomy to have any claim to professional status.

It is best to consider autonomy as a relative concept as even the medical profession is finding its autonomy substantially reduced as government and the new managers of the NHS have imposed strict limits on expenditure, wanting to see value for money and clinical effectiveness. The limited amounts of money available for the NHS coupled with the market economy introduced in the 1980s have led to rationing which, in turn, has reduced the freedom of doctors to prescribe drugs and treatments. If health purchasers will not pay for certain drugs to be prescribed on the NHS, medical autonomy is obviously compromised. The evidence-based practice movement also seeks to challenge the freedom of doctors to do as they wish. Doctors can no longer justify their actions with vague references to 'clinical judgement' as medical practice is increasingly being challenged by the requirement to produce evidence in justification of that practice.

The question of autonomy was at the heart of an interesting discussion by Dent and Burtney (1997) as these authors looked at the concept of professional segmentation. They draw upon the literature to argue that nursing has traditionally consisted of four segments:

❑ 'New managers'. This group originated with the expansion of nursing management in the early 1970s and, although significantly reduced by the reorganizations of the NHS in the 1980s, still constitutes a significant body of nurses.
❑ 'New professionals'. These nurses were keen to extend their roles and took advantage of opportunities offered by the old extended role of the nurse guidelines (see Chapter 5) and the *Scope of Professional Practice* document (UKCC, 1992). Typically they became clinical nurse specialists.
❑ 'The rank and file'. This group is content to work in traditional roles within a medically-dominated hierarchy.
❑ 'The academic professionalizers'. This latter group have tried to develop increased autonomy for nursing based upon nursing theory rather than medical dominance.

Dent and Burtney (1997) use the dramatic growth in the number of practice nurses as a case study of how these four segments have evolved, citing evidence they obtained from interviewing a small number of practice nurses ($n=12$) in two Midlands towns. They consider that practice nurses are developing in four ways, which correspond to the four segments described above. In the same order they are:

❑ Managers and coordinators of care.
❑ Practice Nurse Type I who has actively extended her role by taking on new tasks delegated by GPs, such as nurse-run asthma clinics.
❑ Practice Nurse Type II who has not taken the initiative in extending her role, rather she has remained largely passive and content to do whatever the GP asks.
❑ Nurse practitioners who have sought real autonomy, developing a new role that is more in partnership with the GP.

The most telling point made by Dent and Burtney is that this explosion in practice nurse activity during the 1990s came about as a result of medical sponsorship stimulated by the 1990 GP Contract. There is an obvious analogy with hospital nursing as again it was the impact of the New Deal for Junior Doctors that triggered the growth of a range of new nursing roles. The 'managers' and 'rank and file' remain but the growth in clinical nurse specialists has been followed by the development of increasingly autonomous nurse practitioners who are breaking radical new ground in hospital health care.

The nurse practitioners identified in both primary and hospital health care as the fourth new segment of nursing, the academic professionalizers, only came about as a result of medical sponsorship. It took the new GP contract in 1990 and the impact of the New Deal on availability of junior doctors to stimulate medicine to look to nursing for solutions to health care problems. Medicine did not do this initially because it felt nursing should be given more autonomy and responsibility for health care. This speaks volumes for the degree of autonomy that nursing enjoys and destroys the notion that nursing is a profession because it has the attribute of autonomy.

This discussion of Keogh's paper suggests that the trait approach to defining nursing as a profession lacks validity as most of the attributes claimed for professionalism do not stand up to scrutiny in a nursing context. Perhaps the biggest mismatch is not even mentioned by Keogh and that is the issue of financial reward, a key point where nursing clearly fails the test as a profession. Nursing is not alone in this regard as groups such as teachers, social workers and the various health therapists claim professional status but also suffer from low levels of remuneration, even though their practitioners have higher academic qualifications than nurses (these groups all have degree level education). Consideration of the high and low paid 'professions' suggests there are two key differences. The low paid professions are predominantly female compared to the male-dominated higher paid professions and, while the low paid professions only became organized and 'professionalized' after the state became large scale employers of such people, the higher paid professionals, such as lawyers and doctors, became organized at a time when the state did not employ them, therefore, they were able to exert substantial control over the market for their services and hence assure high rates of remuneration. The problem affecting nurses, teachers and others is that due to their status as employees of the state, they do not have control over the market as the other groups, they have to accept whatever the state will pay.

Alternative views of professionalism

The preceding section consisted of a point by point rebuttal of the validity of the trait approach to professionalism, not withstanding which it is still widely accepted by many nurses who consider themselves professionals as a result. Unfortunately, when questioned as to what they consider 'a professional nurse' to be, none out of a sample of 156 highly educated Australian nurses could give an answer (Coulon *et al.*, 1996). All that these nurses could say was that the term professional was an all encompassing theme indicating the highest standards of care and general excellence in nursing. A similar exercise in the UK might well produce a similar result indicating that nurses are unable actually to articulate what they mean by a professional nurse. This calls into question the validity of the concept of 'a professional nurse'.

There are more fundamental criticisms of the trait approach, however. Parkin (1995) points out two of them; traits are derived from professions rather than a separate theoretical framework. They are therefore tautological and as much use as describing a strawberry by saying it is strawberry coloured or a banana by saying it is banana shaped. Neither of these statements would be much use in helping an Inuit Indian, who had never seen these items before, to recognize a strawberry or banana. Porter (1992) has observed that given the lack of an objective framework from which any list of traits can be derived, who is to say that any one set of traits is the correct description of a profession? There are, therefore, multiple definitions, as any combination of traits can be assembled to describe a profession. This of course is because the traits are derived from the professions themselves rather than an outside frame of reference. Parkin's other telling point is that traits depict professional ideology rather than reality. Descriptions of traits come from within the professions, therefore, they represent the way members of such groups would like to be seen by the public. They are unlikely to cite traits such as incompetence, arrogance or a tendency to commit murder, fraud or adultery which, as we know, have been associated with members of both the legal and medical professions from time to time (and of course nursing).

The suggestion that certain professions are highly paid because of their ability to control the market for their services opens up a new way of thinking about professionalism which is the opposite of the altruistic functionalist perspective. Professions may be seen as groups of workers carving out occupational niches in the labour market for which they claim sole competence and, therefore, eliminate all competition, ensuring maximum prestige and financial rewards (Bilton, 1987). This has nothing to do with public service and everything to do with power and money. Seen from this perspective, the attributes of selection and self-regulation are merely a means to eliminate competition and insulate the profession from public accountability. Members of the general public are always in a minority on bodies such as the UKCC or GMC and therefore have little influence over disciplinary matters. Professionalism is therefore a legal monopoly on practice which uses altruism as a means of justifying the high levels of reward that members of a profession enjoy. Altruism is therefore a smokescreen concealing the sort of closed shop that was made illegal in British industry a decade ago under the Thatcher Government! You may feel that is a rather extreme statement but it merits serious debate because membership of a professional organization (equivalent to a trades union) is a compulsory requirement to be employed in a range of professions such as medicine and law. The altruistic counter-argument is that such membership is a guarantee of competence and ethical practice which protects the public and, in most cases, that is true, but there is a small but significant number of cases where clearly this has not been the case.

Salvage (1992) offered an analysis of nursing consistent with this sceptical view of professionalism. In her view, professional status involved power and politics and, as nursing lacked power, it would never achieve professional status. In Salvage's view nursing has been dominated by medicine and, as it is a predominantly female work force, it is associated with perceptions of low status, menial work that anybody can do. As a result nursing lacks any marketable scarcity value being dismissed as merely 'women's work'. The opposition to affording nurses a university education as a matter of right supports Salvage's contention as if anybody can 'do nursing' why do people need a university degree to become nurses? The saddest part of that rhetorical question is that many of the people asking it are nurses themselves. By taking that point of view they enormously devalue their own occupation and personal worth.

Professionalism can be seen therefore as a crude (and often successful) strategy to manipulate the labour market. This less than flattering notion of professionalism has been further explored in relation to nursing by Davies (1996a) who used the analogy of a cloak. To her, professionalism was something to hide behind. It therefore concealed practice from the gaze of the general public. She also pointed out that the cloak was symbolic of an old-fashioned Victorian gentleman's way of life, which made the analogy even stronger. To Davies, professionalism is bound up in gender stereotypes and the traditional professions are marked by the male characteristics of cold detachment (as opposed to engagement), control of self and others (as opposed to empowerment), competition (as opposed to collaboration) and above all the pursuit of power over others. Professionalism is therefore defined exclusively by male characteristics, consequently it is no coincidence that predominantly female groups such as nurses should find it so difficult to gain recognition as a profession. Traditional professionalism is therefore an 'outdated and male tailored garment' (Davies, 1996a) to which nursing should not aspire. Rather, Davies (1996b) argues for a new vision of professionalism which breaks free from gender bias and involves:

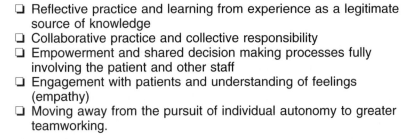

❏ Reflective practice and learning from experience as a legitimate source of knowledge
❏ Collaborative practice and collective responsibility
❏ Empowerment and shared decision making processes fully involving the patient and other staff
❏ Engagement with patients and understanding of feelings (empathy)
❏ Moving away from the pursuit of individual autonomy to greater teamworking.

The challenge posed by Davies is even more fundamental than whether nursing is a profession or not as she challenges the very concept of professionalism as an outdated, male-dominated and literally man-made institution. Groucho Marx once famously said 'I would not want to belong to a club that would have me as a member'. Perhaps nursing should stop striving to belong to the 'Professionals' club on the grounds that it is not the sort of club to which we should belong and, in any case, the entry rules are so constructed that any predominantly female group would automatically be 'black-balled' and, therefore, never gain admission.

Davies' work shifts the debate onto completely new ground as she is arguing with great conviction that nursing is wasting its time pursuing the holy grail of traditional professional status. There is substantial support for her views in the literature even if not in the wider world of nursing where the assumption remains that nursing is a profession. Nursing has pursued several routes towards professional status with marked lack of success, however. Porter (1992) has described how nursing has tried to match itself up against the so called 'trait theory' of professionalism and failed for all the reasons we have discussed already. He also sees the growth of managerialism in nursing, which was spawned by the Salmon Reforms in the 1970s, as evidence of an alternative route to professional status. It was almost as if nursing was saying because we have this extensive managerial pyramid we must be a profession, despite the fact that few nurse managers had any advanced training in management and most had lost contact with clinical nursing. The notion of the nurse as patient advocate is another initially North American route to professionalism, however, in practice, this role is more of a theoretical ideal than reality. This issue will be discussed in more detail on p. 101. Another North American cul de sac identified by Porter was the road to diagnostic autonomy. This began with the nursing process and the illogical insistence that nurses were not to write down a medical diagnosis as a patient problem but either invent some bizarre tautology that nobody understood or write down a statement that could only be called a statement of the blindingly obvious. This former option led to the development of the language of nursing diagnosis which, fortunately, has not been imported to the UK. The development of a clinical elite (clinical nurse specialists and latterly nurse practitioners) is seen by Porter as the final attempt at achieving professional status and is consistent with the process of segmentation described by Dent and Burtney (1997) on p. 42.

The problem with this latter approach is that it leaves behind some 90% of Registered Nurses and sees nursing as rather like an iceberg, the 'professionals' being the tip that can be seen while the vast majority of nurses form an unprofessional underclass, the 'rank and file' of Dent and Burtney's segmentation argument. This will of course lead to yet another cleavage within the ranks of nursing as the clinical elite part company from the rest. The trouble is that the rest are already deeply divided among themselves as Health Visitors, Midwives and Nurses all see themselves as different, while the community/hospital divide is compounded by splits into mental health, children's nursing and a multitude of other client groups. Porter's conclusion is hard to argue with. Nursing should abandon these various attempts to achieve professional status and instead concentrate on being nurses, a skilled and invaluable occupational group who define themselves by what they do rather than trying artificially to achieve status defined by others' rules. This conclusion is consistent with the views of Davies (1996).

Deprofessionalizing nursing

Consideration of arguments such as those above leads to the suggestion that what nursing should really be concerned with is 'deprofessionalization' which Haug (1975) describes as the erosion of monopoly over knowledge, the questioning of autonomy and authority and challenges to status. This is exactly the agenda mapped out by Celia Davies (1996) some 20 years later with reference to nursing. If patients are to be seen as partners in care and educated to care for themselves, knowledge cannot be seen as anybody's monopoly. Knowledge must be shared with patients and it must also be shared between health carers. The expanding skills repertoire of nurse practitioners involves learning techniques of examination and history taking which, up until very recently, were exclusively confined to medicine, another monopoly which is now being eroded.

Questioning autonomy leads into sharing the responsibility for care between health staff and with the patient and family. This was a key theme running through the first two chapters when the concept of care was explored. The issue of authority is closely linked to autonomy and also accountability, as nurses cannot be held accountable for care without the authority to do what they think is right. Authority at present largely rests with medicine and the new breed of general managers. If clinical governance is to be anything other than another trendy catch phrase that will be forgotten in a few years, the authority held by managers has to be questioned and devolved back to clinicians in order that they can be truly accountable. In this context 'clinicians' does not mean doctors only, but all staff involved in health care and, ultimately, authority needs to be given back to the patient in order that he or she may have more control over their care.

The challenge to status goes right to the heart of the matter of course. Look in any hospital car park if you want to understand status. A logical approach might say that lone female staff who had to come and go from work after dark and late at night would have parking spaces reserved immediately outside the well lit main entrance for their own safety and security. However, as we know, those places are reserved for consultants and senior managers while nurses and radiographers are usually left to fend for themselves in the remote and darker recesses of the car park! This is status at work and is the sort of thinking that permeates the whole health system. If status were judged upon the amount of contact the patient had with different groups and how important their presence was perceived to be, then medicine would be some way down the league table and management firmly rooted at the bottom.

Deprofessionalization is therefore about reversing our concern for traditional professional status and returning to a greater service ideal. In health this means rehumanizing care and making patients better informed with a more meaningful patient–practitioner relationship based upon partnership, equality and trust (Parkin, 1996). The notion of engaging the patient was seen to be fundamental to care in the first chapter. The deprofessionalization thesis therefore may have more to offer nursing than the traditional professional model. In the next chapter we shall explore the UKCC *Scope of Professional Practice* document and its implications for current practice. At the heart of this document lies the tension between nurses performing tasks which doctors delegate to them (extended roles) or expanding their practice in a collaborative manner, involving new roles and skills which they feel would benefit patients. The extended role involving delegation of tasks by doctors is consistent with the traditional view of professions as dominant powerful groups controlling and regulating practice from a position of monopoly power. Role expansion by nurses, *in response to patient need*, challenges that monopoly and ultimately the authority upon which it rests making the *Scope of Professional Practice* a potentially revolutionary, or downright dangerous document, depending upon your point of view. The debate about professionalism therefore underpins much of what follows in the next chapter.

Summary

In this chapter we started out with a conventional view of professionalism to which many nurses probably subscribe. The statutory body for nursing (UKCC) also assumes that nursing is a profession as shown by the frequent use of the word 'professional' in its many publications. However, we have seen that 'professionalism' as a concept is open to serious critique on the grounds that it is an out-dated, male-dominated concept into which groups such as nurses do not readily fit. Rather than expend a great deal of effort striving for professional status as defined by tradition and groups such as medicine and the law, perhaps nursing would be better served developing a new occupational model. Nursing should be looking to the future and reflecting upon its core value of caring which leads to viewing patients as partners with whom we should be involved and engaged, rather than passive recipients of our privileged 'expert' knowledge. Individual nurses certainly need to reflect upon what they understand by the term 'professional' and consider whether they want to attach that title to their occupation given the critique of the term developed by various authors cited in this chapter. Nursing might be well served by talking to other groups such as teachers, social workers and the ironically named 'PAMS' in order to develop a consensus around a new view of professionalism, divorced from the masculine bias inherent in the traditional approach and appropriate for staff who are working in caring environments with dependent individuals well into the next century.

References

Benner, P. (1984). *From Novice to Expert*. Menloe Pk: Addison Wesley.

Bilton, A. (1987). *Introductory Sociology*. London: Macmillan Educational.

Coulon, L., Mok, M., Krause, K. and Anderson, M. (1996). The pursuit of excellence in nursing care: what does it mean? *Journal of Advanced Nursing*, **24**, 817–826.

Crouch, S. (1996). Professionals; myth or reality? *Nursing Management*, **3**, 6, 12–13.

Cumberlege (1986). *Community Nursing Review Neighbourhood Nursing: A focus for Care*, London: HMSO.

Davies, C. (1996a). Cloaked in a tattered illusion. *Nursing Times*, **92**, 45, 44–46.

Davies, C. (1996b). A new vision of professionalism. *Nursing Times*, **92**, 46, 54–56.

Dent, M. and Burtney, E. (1997). Changes in practice nursing: professionalism, segmentation and sponsorship. *Journal of Clinical Nursing*, **6**, 355–363.

Fletcher, J. (1997). Do nurses really care? Some unwelcome findings from recent research and enquiry. *Journal of Nursing Management*, **5**, 43–50.

Ford, P. and Walsh, M. (1994). *New Rituals for Old; Nursing Through the Looking Glass*. Oxford: Butterworth-Heinemann.

Haralambos, M. and Holborn, M. (1995). *Sociological Themes and Perspectives* (4th edn). London: Collins Educational.

Haug, M. (1975). The deprofessionalisation of everyone? *Sociological Focus*, **8**, 3, 197–213.

Keogh, J. (1997). Professionalization of nursing development, difficulties and solutions. *Journal of Advanced Nursing*, **25**, 302–308.

Parkin, P. (1995). Nursing the future: a re-examination of the professionalisation thesis in the light of some recent developments. *Journal of Advanced Nursing*, **21**, 561–567.

Porter, S. (1992). The poverty of professionalisation : a critical analysis of strategies for the occupational advancement of nursing. *Journal of Advanced Nursing*, **17**, 720–726.

Salvage, J. (1992). The New Nursing: empowering patients or empowering nurses. In: Robinson, J. (ed.) *Policy Issues in Nursing*. Milton Keynes: OU Press, pp. 9–23.

Shaw, G.B. (1907). *Dramatic Opinons and Essays*, Vol II.

UKCC (1992). *Code of Professional Conduct*. London: UKCC.

UKCC (1992). *The Scope of Professional Practice*. London: UKCC.

CHAPTER 4

Expanding the scope of practice

Wishing me like to one more rich in hope,
Featur'd like him, like him with friends possess'd
Desiring this man's art and that man's scope
With what I most enjoy contented least

William Shakespeare, *Sonnets no. 29.*

Introduction

Shakespeare was writing his sonnets several centuries before the UKCC published their *Scope of Professional Practice* document (UKCC, 1992), however, the debate that has surrounded the whole issue of nursing role expansion echoes Shakespeare's words of unrequited love. Shakespeare's hero starts off by cursing his fate as an outcast, hence his wish to be like '... one more rich in hope'. The declining morale of nursing in the 1990s suggests that nurses too feel outcasts, unloved and unlistened to in the corridors of power, possessed of few friends, and therefore envious of others who have much more power and professional status and consequently hope for a better future. There are many critics who would say nursing has been trying to copy medicine, seeing nurses expanding their roles very much as desiring the doctor's art. Typical of this argument is the view of Castledine (1995), who disparagingly talks of the '... the curiosity and desire of some nurses to pursue a more technical and medical approach to health care' as leading to the development of the nurse practitioner movement which he then dismisses as an obstacle to the growth of specialist nursing. Whether nursing develops its own future role and practice or follows in the footsteps of medicine is one of the key debates about the whole future of nursing and the UKCC Scope document lies at the heart of that debate.

The final line of the excerpt quoted above may reflect the feelings of many nurses today. They came into nursing because they thought they would enjoy it and many actually did for a while, but now they are indeed 'contented least' as plummeting morale and overwork have taken their toll. It is a very uncomfortable feeling to be most unhappy with something that once gave you great pleasure, yet that is how many nurses feel today. There is probably a link between this discontent and nurses seeking to expand their scope of practice by looking at the art of others.

This chapter will draw in the arguments about professionalism from Chapter 3 and look at the tension between nurses trying to expand their roles because they feel it is the right thing to do for the patient and those having their roles extended for them by medical delegation or the need for medical substitution. These are the issues strangely captured in Shakespeare's words and, as we shall see at the end of this chapter, the sonnet does have a positive outcome in the end from which nurses can take heart.

The extended role of the nurse

It is worth looking back at the situation before the UKCC *Scope of Professional Practice* document was published in order to appreciate the background to the present debate about role expansion. Many doctors actually seem unaware of the fundamental changes that have occurred since 1992 and still think in terms of nurses 'extending' their roles in accordance with the pre-1992 guidelines which placed medicine in a very dominant position. It is important at the outset to be precise about terminology and remember that the phrase 'extended role' has a specific meaning as it relates to the Department of Health Circular issued in 1977 which governed policy in this area until 1992. The origins of the 1977 guidance (DoH) were to be found in the realization during the 1970s that, as medical technology dramatically advanced, registered nurses were increasingly being called upon to carry out tasks for which their training had not formally prepared them. Understandably there was a growing concern that such practice should be safe and controlled rather than taking place in an *ad hoc* fashion. The result was a departmental working party, which met for 3 years before coming out with the 1977 circular. The main points in the guidance were as follows:

❏ Nurses may extend their role only in an emergency or as a result of delegation by doctors
❏ Delegation should occur when the doctors are assured of the nurse's competence to perform the task
❏ Training should be given to the nurse with whom the employer is satisfied
❏ The task is one that is recognized as being appropriate for a nurse to perform
❏ The nurse agrees to perform the task
❏ The nurse is liable in law if he or she fails to carry out the task when he or she should or if he or she is incompetent in carrying out the task.

It became standard practice that once a nurse had shown competence to perform a task, a certificate of competence for that task was issued.

Taking these points one by one, the reader is struck by the dominant position occupied by medicine as it is the doctor's decision which new tasks will be *delegated* to nurses and also whether they are competent to perform them. There is no 'professional autonomy' here as clearly medicine is in control of nursing. Only those rather tedious tasks of which doctors wanted to be rid, such as giving intravenous injections of antibiotics or taking blood would be delegated to nurses. There is little scope for the nurse to take the initiative and decide how he or she would like to extend his or her role in response to patient need.

The second point assumes that doctors are competent in the performance of clinical tasks, or else there would be no justification for letting them be the arbiters of the nurse's capability. Discussion of this point with many experienced post-registration students provides much anecdotal evidence to question the validity of that assumption. The old medical dictum of 'see one, do one, teach one' hardly infused the average staff nurse with confidence when an SHO was attempting to assess his or her competence as it rather questioned the depth of experience of many doctors. It also raises the question of whether being judged competent once is a reliable indicator of a person's competence 5 or 10 years later. The same argument can be applied to passing the driving test of course.

Standards of training for extended role tasks were left to each individual employer which, in practical terms, led to a great deal of variability as the number of employers of nurses runs into thousands within the NHS and private sectors. There were no national standards and the situation was made worse when one employer refused to recognize the certificate of competence of another. This led to nurses embarking on a never-ending paper chase whenever they moved jobs in order to collect a whole new file of competency certificates (which usually only proved they were judged competent on one occasion, by a standard which was not recognized anywhere else and rarely supported by any evidence). Such a certificate, as we have said, was no proof of competency in 3 or 4 years time as outmoded techniques could linger on for years in the absence of proper continuing education and evidence-based practice. Those Trusts that still keep the certificate of competency system in the belief that it is a successful risk management strategy should consider the serious weaknesses outlined here.

The extended role guidelines stated that a task should be one that was recognized as appropriate for nurses to perform. This begs the obvious question, recognized by whom? The nurse and the patient are the two most important stakeholders in deciding what it is appropriate for a nurse to do yet the DoH Circular made scant reference to either in the decision making process concerning appropriateness. The implicit answer was of course that the doctor should decide what was appropriate which, again, exposes the myth that nursing was a profession by virtue of autonomy in practice, one of the key traits proposed by adherents to the trait theory of professions discussed in Chapter 3. The only active part the nurse had in the whole process was whether he or she agreed to perform the task when given the right to refuse role extension. This was very difficult in practice as immense pressure could be brought to bear by medical staff and senior management together with the implicit threat that if the individual nurse did not take on the new role then the management would find another nurse who would.

The issue of liability came as something of a shock to many nurses who laboured under the misapprehension (as many nurses still do) that in some strange way they 'were covered by their employer'. The issue of vicarious liability will be explored in Chapter 5, but suffice it to say that nurses have always been liable for their actions in law.

Perhaps the most fundamental criticism of this approach to the extended role of the nurse was the way it reduced nursing to a series of tasks. The patient as a whole human being became lost in debates about tasks. Perhaps this is not surprising as we saw in Chapter 2 that up to the 1970s nursing had been task focused and all nursing work was organized on the basis of a hierarchy of tasks which were delegated to different grades of nurses depending upon their technical complexity. Nobody was thinking about the whole person.

There is a fundamental danger for nursing if we only focus on tasks and that danger is just as real today as it was in the days of the 'extended role'. The dangers of a task focus also need to be considered when considering the *Scope of Professional Practice* document, as there are still many people who interpret the Scope document in terms of tasks only. The key point is that if nursing is reduced merely to a series of tasks of varying complexity, there will be budget-focused managers who might consider that they can train other individuals to perform the tasks more cheaply and therefore replace nurses with NVQ trained health technicians. As Mitchell (1997) succinctly puts it, health care staff who define themselves in terms of a series of tasks should prepare for replacement! Mitchell argues that it is better to define nursing in terms of quality, process and the meaningful experience of the consumer as there is no professional practice in carrying out routine assessments ('admitting a patient' or 'doing the obs') and technical procedures (changing a dressing). She goes on to state that if something does not depend upon feedback from the patient and a person (the RN) then having to make a judgement about what to do next does not need an RN to do it. The registered nurse should *respond* to a blood pressure of 80/50, a wound that is obviously infected or a patient talking of suicide with an intervention. If he or she does not, then he or she is certainly negligent and, probably, not fit to hold a nursing qualification.

There are very strong ties with the views advanced about caring in Chapter 1, where a series of nurse authors argued that caring was about interpersonal interaction between nurse and patient. It is in the essence of that 'one to one' that true nursing can be found and this is what separates the care offered by a qualified nurse from that available from a technician. In an extensive study of nursing care, Carr-Hill *et al.* (1992) found that wards with a high proportion of registered nurses offered better quality and more cost effective care than wards with a higher number of health care assistants because the RN was able to react to patient situations, decide what to do next and then do it without having to ask other staff. This is of course exactly the point that Mitchell is making as she also reminds us that the basic reason nurses exist is because patients want nurses to care for them, not technicians in white coats. This is because patients who are ill want to be listened to, treated with respect as an individual in a non-judgemental way and, above all, cared for and helped to deal with the crises that illness produces. This is the vision of what nursing should be outlined in Chapter 1. For the nurse to respond in such an interactive way requires significant levels of authority and autonomy together with a level of education that will support these greater levels of clinical freedom. This underlines the argument in favour of nursing being a graduate entry occupation rather than regressing to the apprenticeship training that preceded the Diploma in HE education that nurses receive today.

Strong support for abandoning task-based definitions of nursing may also be found in the work of Hansten and Washburn (1998). They also argue anybody can be trained to perform a specific task, but it is the ability to recognize patterns of behaviour in the context of a scientific knowledge background and then integrate individual tasks into a coherent package of care that separates the work of the nurse from the technician. According to Hansten and Washburn, the nurse's role is to help the patient navigate his way through the health care system and a moment's pause for reflection will reveal that the first and last person most patients encounter during a period of illness is the nurse. The point could be taken further as the first and last person most individuals encounter in their entire life will hold a nursing/midwifery qualification. The medical profession wisely take care not to define themselves in terms of individual tasks but rather in terms of the diagnostic process and total responsibility for and authority over all treatment offered. This is one of the strategies medicine has used to maintain its monopoly position and largely avoid the danger of being replaced by technicians but, as the discussion later in this chapter on emerging nurse practitioner roles will show, doctors are becoming concerned that they may be replaced by nurses.

The focus of the old extended role guidelines on tasks did nursing a grave disservice in many ways, not least because, apart from making the whole patient invisible, it left nursing open to the predations of cost cutting managers who, only thinking tasks, logically began to think of training cheaper pairs of hands to do those tasks, i.e. health care assistants and technicians. The increasing shortages of nurses that have plagued the NHS in the late 1990s may also lead NHS managers, eager for a quick fix, to think in terms of recruiting health care assistants and technicians who can be trained very quickly and deployed in clinical areas in a fraction of the time it takes to educate an RN. If we allow health care debate to remain bogged down in a 'who does what job' task-focused agenda, nursing and patients will be the losers. Quality health care needs a focus on the interactive process of care, from a point of view that includes the patient.

The scope of professional practice

Although the UKCC published this document in 1992, experience of teaching post-registration courses suggests to me that there are many nurses who are unaware of its contents or who at best only have a hazy notion of the important points that it makes. Many doctors are unaware of its existence and still think about nurses in terms of the 1977 Department of Health circular on the extended role discussed above.

The document draws the practitioner's attention at an early stage to the Code of Conduct whose basic principles underpin Scope. The Code reminds you that the interests of the patient are paramount at all times. The primacy of the patient or what is in the patient's best interests is the fundamental principle that governs practice. You are also expected to improve your knowledge and keep up to date with current practice while acknowledging your limitations in such a way that you do not undertake tasks unless you can perform them in a safe and skilled manner. The UKCC holds you personally accountable for fulfilling these requirements. It is essential to hold on to these key points while reading the following discussion about the Scope document.

The Scope document lists six principles that control the degree to which a practitioner alters their area of practice:

❑ Activities must serve the interests of the patient at all times
❑ The practitioner must have the knowledge and competence to meet the patient's needs
❑ You must acknowledge limitations of knowledge and skill and take steps to remedy any deficits
❑ You must ensure that any expansion in your role is not at the expense of existing practice and always complies with the Code of Conduct
❑ The practitioner must remember his/her personal accountability for all practice
❑ Delegation of work to others must always be done appropriately and in the patient's best interests.

The first of these points requires the nurse to consider whose interests are being served by taking on a new role. If the answer is that the junior doctors would benefit, this is not an adequate reason. The Trust might argue that nurses are cheaper than doctors so getting them to do doctors' work saves money. That again is not a reason that fits the UKCC principles, as the only beneficiary there is the Trust. It is clear though that nurses taking on intravenous work such as blood sampling, drug administration and cannulation can benefit the patient as for example it speeds up treatment or ensures that drug levels in the bloodstream remain within therapeutic levels. However, the nurse should remember the comments of Mitchell (1997) and Hansten and Washburn (1998) for simply performing these tasks in isolation is not nursing. They need to be incorporated within the nursing role in a meaningful way that involves action. When the blood results are rung back from the laboratory the nurse needs to know their significance and whether immediate action is needed or they can be logged in the patient's notes and left for the doctors. The nurse needs to be able to know what a reaction to an intravenous drug dose might look like and what to do if one occurs and be empowered to take appropriate action. It is the completion of a full cycle of care based upon feedback from the initial action that incorporates a new task into holistic nursing care.

If the nurse did not have the knowledge or competence to perform a new role then not only would he or she be in breach of the Code of Conduct, but would also be negligent in the full legal sense of the term (see Chapter 5) and personally liable for the consequences of his or her actions. It is obvious good sense therefore to acknowledge your limitations, however this may not be so easy for two reasons. First, the nurse might be under considerable pressure to perform tasks and roles with inadequate preparation and find it very difficult to say no for fear of losing his or her job. Crouch (1996) is concerned that nurses who expand their roles without adequate education are not only placing themselves in a very exposed position but are also denigrating nursing as they are merely confirming the doctor's loyal handmaiden stereotype. The debate surrounding the nurse practitioner role is illustrative of this problem; for while there is an excellent honours degree programme available from the RCN Institute and franchising universities to prepare nurses for nurse practitioner posts, many others find themselves thrust into a variety of 'nurse practitioner' roles with little more than a few days in-house training to prepare them. Such nurses are very exposed and the safety of their practice has to be seriously questioned.

There is also a more subtle problem involved in role expansion which can best be summed up by asking the question, 'How do you know what you don't know?' You may think your practice is competent or that you have the knowledge base to carry out certain tasks and interpret patient feedback to plan what to do next but, supposing you are wrong, how will you know except when something goes badly wrong? This points out the importance of nurses having both adequate formal post-registration education and access to good in-service training. However, more is needed than education and reflective practice is widely acknowledged as having a major role to play in professional development. Authors such as James and Clarke (1994) have, however, challenged the assumption that reflective practice is the panacea for all nursing's problems, calling for research to evaluate its impact. Wilkinson (1999) has rightly pointed out that many nurses have only a superficial knowledge of reflection and that there are significant ethical problems posed by reflection in terms of the person's own self-concept and the confidentiality of the information being reviewed.

Other strategies which can help the nurse include clinical supervision, peer review and good teamwork involving medical colleagues, all of which require the nurse to admit he or she is not sure or does not know and crucially to accept constructive suggestions for the improvement of practice in a non-threatening supportive environment. Sadly, such an environment has been conspicuous by its absence in the 1990s as a result of the Conservative Government NHS reforms which established a market in health care and led to a new breed of 'macho' general managers. This problem is exacerbated by the fact that some nurses are perhaps not as good as they could be at taking *constructive* criticism or recognizing their weaknesses. There are many reasons why this should be including the culture of the NHS, fear of criticism and the destructive experiences that some nurses have had.

The Labour administration, which took over in 1997, took a fresh view of the NHS and one of its innovations was to introduce the notion of clinical governance in its White Paper of 1997 (DoH, 1997). This concept was rather vaguely defined, but the principle behind it was to give more responsibility back to clinicians as a way of improving the quality of services delivered. In the following year the Government introduced their white paper 'A First Class Service, Quality in the NHS' (DoH, 1998) which came up with a more precise definition. Clinical governance was:

> 'A framework through which NHS organisations are accountable for continuously improving the quality of their services and safeguarding high standards of care by creating an environment in which excellence in clinical care will flourish.'

Scott (1998) observed that monitoring the quality of care and staff support is an essential element of clinical governance. There has to be a shift away from a defensive culture of blame to one of openness in clinical practice with true multidisciplinary cooperation if the idea is to work. However, as Scott points out, this will take time to develop. Although still in the developmental stages, it is possible that the clinical governance agenda will provide a more favourable context within which nursing staff may develop their roles and honestly reflect upon the quality of their care through audit and review.

There is one final problem with the exhortation that nurses must take steps to remedy their deficits and that is continuing professional education and access to formal courses. The former was meant to be addressed by PREP, but recently published research shows that nurses have a detached and disinterested attitude towards PREP, regarding it as merely another UKCC imposition. This research also questions the value to practice of many of the courses that nurses attend (Scott, 1999). Many nurses find access to formal courses very difficult as places are rationed; time off from the clinical area is hard to obtain; they are often expected to pay the full fees themselves; and the geographical distribution of courses is such that even if all the above problems can be overcome, the nurse may find attendance at the course involves a round trip of over 100 miles.

Investment in continuing education for nurses needs to be made a new priority for the NHS. If the clinical governance agenda is to be meaningfully implemented there must be an emphasis upon life-long learning and professional development programmes (Wilson, 1998) which, fortunately, means that the goals of the UKCC and the Government coincide. In order to improve access to courses, the university sector needs to invest in video-conferencing facilities which can dramatically reduce the amount of travelling part-time students have to do and make education far more accessible, particularly in rural areas.

An alternative to course-based education is offered by project-based, practice development work. This may produce more positive results than merely relying on staff attending courses as there is no guarantee that what is learnt on a course can be translated into practice. There are many contextual barriers to be overcome before change can occur and staff need constructive facilitation to develop practice. McCormack (1999) has proposed a powerful model of practice development which sees the outcome as a function of evidence, context and facilitation. In other words, simply sending a nurse on a course may help the person gain some evidence, but that on its own will not develop practice as it pays no attention to the context in which the nurse works or the need for facilitation to help change practice. NHS Trust education-purchasing consortia should therefore purchase practice development work as well as courses from their local universities. A mix of education and practice development project work is essential if nurses are to be able to comply with their Code of Conduct, the *Scope of Professional Practice* and the demands being placed upon them by employers in response to the rapidly changing health care environment.

The Scope document rightly reminds nurses that developing new roles must not compromise existing practice. As time cannot be stretched, except in the bizarre world of Einstein's Relativity Theory, the nurse only has a fixed number of hours to work with in any shift. Nurses do not have spare time while on duty. If new roles and tasks are to be incorporated into the nurse's everyday work, something has to give. Some existing aspects of practice have to be set aside to make room for the new work for it will be folly to try to take on more and more work within a fixed time period. This could lead to unsafe and unsatisfactory practice (breaching the Code of Conduct) or the nurse would eventually suffer burnout through stress and overwork. This is where the next principle for role expansion comes into play for, as nurses set aside work in order to make room for new tasks and roles, they must ensure that the work set aside is still completed, because if patient care becomes fragmented or incomplete, they have failed to comply with Scope and the Code of Professional Conduct. The nurse therefore has to work smarter and learn to delegate.

It may be that this is a good time to review all the things that a nurse actually does, for it may be that some things are only done because they always have been and could easily be discontinued without harm to the patient. Other things could be done differently and by working smarter the nurse can save time. For example do you really need all those patients on 4-hourly observations? If patients were responsible for self-medication how much time would that save? The nurse might also consider the amount of time spent writing in nursing care plans and consider the introduction of critical pathways which could save considerable amounts of time while improving multidisciplinary communication. It would be a mistake to assume that nothing can be done to reduce the pressure on nurses' time. Perhaps the NHS has been too obsessed with cost cutting rather than looking at how to save the time of the existing staff in order that it can be better used. That is a more quality-focused route to improving efficiency.

When all time saving options have been explored, there may still be inadequate time for the nurse to take on new roles, which then raises the issue of delegation to others, including the patient and their family. The

Scope document reminds the nurse to consider how appropriate it is to delegate to an individual and, as we shall shortly see, it has a lot more to say about delegation.

The final key principle in Scope concerns personal accountability for all aspects of practice whether expanded roles or not and this will be considered in detail in Chapter 6.

The UKCC Scope document, having established these six principles, then goes on to make a very important statement:

> '. . . it is the Council's principles for practice rather than certificates for tasks which should form the basis for adjustments to the scope of professional practice.'
> UKCC (1992) Scope of Professional Practice(p. 9.)

This statement was aimed at moving nursing fundamentally away from the certification mentality that characterized the former extended role concept and, in effect, made nurses arbiters of their own competence and practice. Despite this document, many Trusts still adhere to certificates of competency in the belief that this constitutes an effective risk management strategy. The fallacies inherent in this argument have already been discussed (p. 52); meanwhile, reliance on certificates undermines the potential beneficial impact of the *Scope of Professional Practice* document. This has to be contrasted with many areas of primary health care where nurse practitioners have dramatically expanded their role without embarking on a paper chase and with other progressive hospital trusts who have moved forward with the spirit of the UKCC Scope paper. The key issue is perhaps whether managers are prepared to *trust* nurses to be arbiters of their own competence, although there is no easy way around the awkward question of 'How do you know what you do not know?' The move away from certificates also requires managers to move away from seeing nursing simply in terms of a series of tasks and, instead, to see nursing as 'joined up care', whereby the nurse delivers a holistic package of care to an individual patient for which he or she is prepared to be held accountable. When care is seen in this way certificates become redundant.

It is however important that nurses do accept accountability for their actions. Reference has already been made to the 'Are we covered for that?' mentality which sees somebody else as always taking the ultimate responsibility for what the nurse does. The nurse must insist on adequate preparation and education for any expanded role before undertaking it (Hunt and Wainwright, 1994), however much pressure there may be. A crucial example is the plan to roll out the NHS Direct scheme whereby nurses will be offering advice to the general public about an infinite range of health problems. Although they will be assisted by computer software, this will only go so far and ultimately the nurse's own knowledge and skill will play a key part. Training has to consist of more than an intensive package to familiarize the nurse with the software. Research by the author (Walsh, 1999) indicates that common areas of enquiry at a pilot NHS Direct site include childhood illnesses, trauma, pharmacology and mental health problems. While a nurse with a background in Accident and Emergency nursing might be very comfortable dealing with questions concerning trauma, it is more doubtful whether he or she can deal safely and effectively with calls concerning childhood immunizations, the possibility of a drug interaction, or from a distressed person with mental health problems, unless there has been effective training and education which is appropriate for his/her needs. If the nurse falls back on a safety first approach of repeatedly telling the caller to contact their GP or attend A&E as he or she is not sure, then there is no point in NHS Direct, as one of the main points of the service is to reduce the demand on GPs and A&E departments!

The issue of delegation is explored later in the Scope document which reminds registered nurses that they are always accountable for the assessment, planning and standards of care carried out by staff to whom they have delegated care. This includes health care assistants and also students who must not be allowed to work beyond their level of competence. Health care assistants should be seen as full members of the health care team in order to ensure good teamwork and coordinated care. The nurse therefore may find that he or she has to delegate work to health care assistants in order to comply with the Scope document's principle that role expansion must not compromise existing care, however he or she remains accountable at all times for the care delegated. It is necessary therefore to know your health care assistants well so that you do know the limits of their ability. Good training opportunities for health care assistants will enhance their contribution in addition to treating them as full team members, which is of course what the Scope says you should be doing anyway. Some nurses may find themselves uncomfortable with the idea that they are being held accountable for the work of others, but that is the reality of the situation. The health care assistant remains responsible in law for their actions, however, even though the nurse is professionally accountable to the UKCC.

The document offers a practical way forward that allows nurses to expand their practice in response to patient need rather than managerial and medical convenience. However, there are problems of which nurses must be aware, the first of which is the key issue of whether nurses can assess their own competence and therefore know the limits of their practice. This issue is not seen as a problem by professions such as medicine who do not have other professional groups overseeing their practice, consequently it would be illogical to assert that nursing should be policed by medicine, which in effect was the arrangement under the extended role guidelines. However, the tragic events involving the cardiac surgery unit at the Bristol Royal Infirmary have highlighted the need for internal monitoring and control of standards of practice by various health care groups. Audit and evidence-based practice are powerful safeguards against nurses straying into areas which lie beyond their competency, while clinical supervision, reflective practice and peer review will provide continual feedback on how well the nurse is performing. The National Institute of Clinical Excellence (NICE), which is being set up to promote the use of evidence-based guidelines, could play a vital role in ensuring that nurses, as well as doctors, stay within the bounds of effectiveness. Ultimately, however, taking responsibility for your own practice is a key component of clinical governance.

Cynics might note that the changes associated with the *Scope of Professional Practice* have coincided with the New Deal for junior hospital doctors resulting in substantial reductions in their working hours. At the same time, General Practice is facing problems with recruitment. A greater willingness on the part of the Department of Health to give nurses more freedom over their practice might have more to do with resolving medical staffing problems than recognizing the value and status of nurses. This need not be a problem as long as nurses are aware of the possible motivation that lies behind recent changes for, whatever the reason, nurses are being offered a much better framework within which to expand their practice than the old extended role. The danger is, though, that nurses may just be viewed as cheap medical substitutes, which they are not. Such a perspective is clearly at odds with the thinking that lies behind the Scope document and maintains nursing's subservient position with regard to medicine. The expanded role of the nurse is about nursing deciding how to expand its role in line with patient need rather than being told to pick up the boring bits of medicine for which there are insufficient junior doctors to cope.

The NHS has been subject to many reforms and restructuring exercises over the years. A major problem, however, has been that while the structures may be changed, the systems remain the same and, as Dowglass (1999) points out, this incongruency means it is very difficult to change things. If the system remains 'doctors are in charge', no amount of structural change will move nursing practice forward. Trying to implement clinical governance or develop new nursing structures within the context of New Deal and the *Scope of Professional Practice* will therefore only succeed if attention is paid to the systems by which things are achieved, i.e. who decides what nurses will do and how they will do it. (See Chapter 2). This of course requires a significant change of culture in some areas of the NHS.

Nursing expansion will clearly bring it into contact with other groups of health care workers and boundary disputes or turf battles, as they call them in the USA, are possible. Although the boundaries with medicine are the obvious potential conflict zone, radiography has provided a second area of dispute while community nurses may have difficulty deciding where their responsibility ends and the social worker's begins. There is no doubt that the borders with medicine are blurring (Hunt and Wainwright, 1994) and, while this can lead to conflict, it can also lead to a great deal of innovative and creative practice.

Dynamic systems are potentially chaotic; one characteristic of which is that a small disturbance can produce unforeseen, massive consequences, the so-called butterfly effect, after the notion that the flap of a butterfly's wings on a tropical island can eventually lead to a massive hurricane sweeping into the southern states of the USA (Gleick, 1987). The whole subject of chaos theory has recently emerged from scholarly and academic cloisters where it has overturned many conventional ways of thinking about the natural sciences. Chaos theory is now being discussed in relation to a range of behaviours such as the Stock Markets of the world, ecological systems and even human physiology. Dynamic systems can simplistically be defined as those where behaviour in one part depends upon feedback from others in a sensitive way (Cohen and Stewart, 1994). Nursing and medicine both have such characteristics in that changes in one area depend upon changes elsewhere and, by analogy with the natural sciences, could be seen as chaotic, especially at the boundary where they interface. Such boundary conditions are inherently unstable and have been the subject of much scientific study. The analogy with the natural sciences, therefore, suggests that the development of practice at the interface of medicine and nursing is likely to be unpredictable and surprising with small changes today potentially producing major consequences in the future. This makes for interesting and exciting practice development opportunities even if the ride is likely to be somewhat bumpy at times!

The issue of what happens at the boundaries of nursing and medicine has been very much brought into focus by the growth of the nurse practitioner movement, which was made possible in the UK by the *Scope of Professional Practice* document. It is regrettable therefore that the 1990s have been characterized by the unedifiying sight of nursing's professional body (the UKCC) failing to grasp the significance of nurse practitioner development. Comments such as Castledine's infamous dismissal of nurse practitioners as an 'obstacle' to the UKCC's grand plan for specialist nursing, coupled with his comments that they have evolved to '. . . satisfy the curiosity and desire of some nurses to pursue a more technical and medical approach to the subject of health care' (Castledine, 1995), reveal the lack of vision and leadership shown by the UKCC. It is of course so ironic that this should come after the UKCC had the earlier vision and courage to produce the Scope document in the first place. It is almost as if they had let the genie out of the bottle with Scope and then did not know what to do with it. Evidence gathered by Walsh (1999) refutes the assertion that nurse practitioners are only interested in the technical and medical aspects of care as his research has shown that they give a significantly higher priority to the psychosocial dimensions of care than conventional nurses.

The definition of the nurse practitioner role produced by the RCN contradicts the 'mini-doctor' allegation and can be summarized as follows:

The nurse practitioner:

- ❑ Sees patients with undiagnosed and undifferentiated problems
- ❑ Carries out a health assessment using extra skills not normally taught in nursing education to date (this includes history taking and physical examination skills)
- ❑ Makes professionally autonomous decisions for which he or she has sole responsibility
- ❑ Develops a plan of *nursing care* to promote health
- ❑ Provides counselling and health education
- ❑ Screens patients for early signs of illness and risk factors
- ❑ May admit, discharge or refer patients.

This role needs to be supported by appropriate education at honours degree level.

Nurse practitioners are therefore not cheap doctor substitutes and, while research shows that they are very popular with patients and highly appreciated, patients can tell the difference and will chose between the doctor or nurse practitioner depending upon the nature of their condition (Coopers and Lybrand, 1996; Salisbury and Tettersal, 1987; Stilwell *et al.*,1988). They do not therefore constitute a threat to medicine, rather a complementary service that gives patients more choice and allows doctors more time to concentrate on the sort of health problems for which they have a natural preference and the training. The Coopers and Lybrand report (1996) looked at 10 different nurse practitioner projects in a range of settings and their findings were similar to many other evaluative studies. They stated that nurse practitioners gave a different style of service that improved access, reduced waiting times and freed up considerable amounts of medical time. High degrees of patient satisfaction were found as the nurse practitioner services were able to cross both disciplinary boundaries and the primary/secondary healthcare divide while providing health care to previously marginalized groups such as the homeless. The key research question for nurse practitioners is not so much *whether* they are effective but *why* are they so effective? It is likely that these comments can also be applied to other nurses who have expanded their role, but without adopting the nurse practitioner label.

A useful way of conceptualizing what is happening and, at the same time reassuring anxious colleagues in other disciplines, is to think of the field of health care as a space. It can then be viewed in two ways, one of which involves looking out of my window now as I type this chapter. I see a large field of approximately 5 acres surrounded by a drystone wall containing some very windswept and soggy Swaledale sheep. That field has a fixed boundary (the drystone wall), therefore, any small group of those sheep can only expand their grazing at the expense of the other sheep in the field. Seeing health care in that way means that any discipline (such as nursing) can only expand its area of activity at the expense of another as the overall area is fixed and constant. The result will be the friction and disharmony with which we are all familiar and which prevents practice development. The harmful effect on patient care of such interprofessional bickering has frequently been seen by nurses and is described in research by Woroch (1999). She found evidence of information being deliberately withheld by one group of professionals from another while others refused to cooperate with clinical nurse specialists, each time to the detriment of the patient.

However, if we turn to cosmology for another way of thinking, we come across the model of the expanding universe in which space is continually expanding in all directions at once as the millions of galaxies that make up the known universe all rush away from each other. This actually is a better analogy for the universe of health care than the field surrounded by a drystone wall, as the universe of health care is an expanding universe rather than the static 5-acre field. Consider the dramatic changes over the last few decades as new treatments and drugs have become available, the increase in numbers of elderly people living longer, the new diseases and threats to health that have emerged to replace the old dreaded infectious diseases (which may yet be lurking ready to make a comeback at any time). All this in the context of dramatic social change means that the universe of health care is expanding and any discipline can expand its area of activity without affecting the others as this is not a static field, the whole place is expanding! In fact if disciplines did not expand to keep pace with their universe, gaps and holes would start to appear in the fabric of that universe; there would not be a universal health care service and increasing numbers of people would fall down those holes and lose their access to care. No one discipline can cover this whole expanding universe either, it needs expansion and cooperation by all of us.

This cosmological analogy suggests that the expansion of the nursing role is actually necessary to maintain health care access and should not disadvantage any other discipline. Seen in that way, we can view boundaries as exciting places where new developments can occur and cross fertilization of ideas and practice can produce exciting new hybrids. Boundaries should not consist of trenches and barbed wire entanglements and they do not need to be zones of conflict.

There remains a final key issue and that is whether nurses can be held accountable in the way Scope requires when they have so little power. The key principles that make Scope work are that the individual nurse has to stand up and be counted for his or her practice and nurses should be taking the initiative in decisions on practice expansion, rather than leaving such decisions exclusively to the medical profession. A critical social science philosophy therefore has much to offer nursing as it is concerned with making visible systems of oppression and control within societies (McCormack, 1999). Ford and Walsh (1994) have applied a critical social science analysis to nursing, arguing that nurses are a subordinated group, subject to patterns of control which limit their autonomy and hence accountability. An emancipatory agenda is therefore necessary if the full benefits of the *Scope of Professional Practice* are to be realized. The systems by which health care operates will have to change if the structures inherent in the concept of nurse accountability are to work.

Summary

The UKCC *Scope of Professional Practice* (1992) offered nursing an exciting way of moving forward which many nurses have embraced. However, misunderstanding, unimaginative management, the general air of crisis that has affected the NHS since 1992 and the attitudes of some members of the medical profession have held back nursing's development. In order to obtain the full potential benefits of 'Scope', nursing needs to approach role expansion in a structured but flexible way. The following steps are therefore suggested as guidelines:

1   The first point is to establish whether the patient is the main beneficiary of the nurse taking on a new role or task. This is the main criterion so far as the UKCC are concerned

2   A careful search of the evidence base should be carried out in order to ensure best practice is followed. Consideration should be given on how to translate the evidence into a solution that will work in the local context.

3   The education and training required for role expansion should then be ascertained and arrangements made for their delivery.

4   The other staff likely to be affected by the change should be involved in discussion and explanation in order to avoid confusion and possible hostility.

5   The nurse needs to review his or her own workload to ensure existing work does not suffer as a result of the new role and arrangements should be made if work has to be delegated or re-structured.

6   Support networks need to be in place for the nurse such as clinical supervision, peer-group review, practice development supervision. Role expansion can be very stressful.

7   Decisions have to be made about how to evaluate the effect of the changes and data gathered pre-change, for comparison purposes. These need to reflect quality of service as seen by the patient, other health professionals and also costs in order that clinical effectiveness can be assessed.

8   Only when these stages are complete can role expansion and practice change occur. It should be done in such a way that feedback could readily inform the emerging new role, permitting rapid adjustments in practice as necessary.

9   A more formal evaluation and report on progress should follow later on in the development process.

10   The nurse should be aware of the need to market the new role, assuming success, in order that the changes made become permanent.

References

Carr-Hill, R., Dixon, P., Gibbs, I. *et al.* (1992). *Skill Mix and the Effectiveness of Nursing Care.* York: University of York.

Castledine, G. (1995). Defining specialist nursing. *British Journal of Nursing*, **4**, 5, 264–265.

Cohen, J. and Stewart, I. (1994). *The Collapse of Chaos.* New York: Penguin.

Coopers and Lybrand (1996). Nurse Practitioner Evaluation Report. London: HMSO.

Crouch, S. (1996). Professionals – myth or reality? *Nursing Management*, **3**, 6, 12–13.

Department of Health (1977). DoH Circular. *The Extended Role of the Nurse*. London, Department of Health.

DoH (1997). *The New NHS; Modern, Dependable*. London: The Stationery Office.

DoH (1998). *A First Class Service; Improving Quality in the NHS*. London: The Stationery Office.

Dowglass, M. (1999). Practice Development; Managing the Process. Foundation for Nursing Studies 4th Annual Conference of the Professional Practice Development Nurses Forum, Blackpool, 1999.

Ford, P. and Walsh, M. (1994). *New Rituals for Old*. Oxford: Butterworth-Heinemann.

Gleick, J. (1987). *Chaos*. London: Sphere Books.

Hansten, R. and Washburn, M. (1998). Professional practice facts and impact. *American Journal of Nursing*, **98**, 3, 42–45.

Hunt, G. and Wainwright, P. (1994). *Expanding the Role of the Nurse*. Oxford: Blackwell Scientific.

James, C. and Clarke, B. (1994). Reflective practice in nursing; issues and implications for nurse education. *Nurse Education Today*, **14**, 82–90.

McCormack, B. (1999). A Model for Practice Development. Foundation for Nursing Studies 4th Annual Conference of the Professional Practice Development Nurses Forum, Blackpool, 1999.

Mitchell, G. (1997). Reengineered healthcare: why nurses matter. *Nursing Science Quarterly*, **10**, 2, 70–71.

Salisbury, C. and Tettersal, M. (1987). Comparison of the work of a nurse practitioner with that of a general practitioner. *Journal of the Royal College of General Practitioners*, **38**, 314–316.

Scott, A. (1998). Clinical governance relies upon a change in culture. *British Journal of Nursing*, **7**, 16, 940.

Scott, B. (1999). Nurses are detached and not interested in PREP. *Nursing Standard*, **13**, 24, 7.

Stilwell, B., Greenfield, S., Drury, M. and Hull, F. (1988). A nurse practitioner in General Practice; patient perceptions and expectations. *Journal of the Royal College of General Practitioners*, **38**, 503–505.

UKCC (1992). *The Scope of Professional Practice*. London: UKCC.

Walsh, M. (1999.) Staff perceptions of working at an NHS Direct pilot site. Unpublished.

Walsh, M. (1999). Nurses and nurse practitioners' 1: priorities in care. *Nursing Standard*, **13**, 24, 38–42.

Wilkinson, J. (1999). Implementing reflective practice. *Nursing Standard*, **13**, 21, 36–40.

Wilson, J. (1998). Clinical governance. *British Journal of Nursing*, **7**, 16, 985–986.

Woroch, K. (1999). Rivalries are causing barrier to learning. *Nursing Standard*, **13**, 22, 9.

CHAPTER 5

Legal considerations in expanding the scope of professional practice

'Ignorance of the law excuses no man; not that all men know the law, but because 'tis an excuse all men will plead and no man can tell how to confute him'

John Selden (1689) *Table Talk*, p.99 Law

Introduction

John Selden's famous dictum has obvious implications for nursing, especially when nursing is seeking to expand its boundaries of practice within an increasingly litigious society. In the preceding chapter we saw how the UKCC document *The Scope of Professional Practice* (1992) offered nurses a real opportunity to move away from the medical dominance of the old and discredited 'extended role' concept. Experience in teaching nurses about the implications of Scope has shown me that many nurses are very anxious about whether they are 'covered' to carry out new tasks and develop new roles. When questioned as to what they mean by 'covered', the answers forthcoming from nurses are often vague and unsure but usually relate to some notion of protection from being sued if things go wrong. Sadly there is often a great deal of misunderstanding and confusion surrounding nurses' knowledge of the law and such ignorance will, as Selden pointed out over 300 years ago, be no defence in the event of a nurse finding herself involved in legal proceedings. This chapter does not set out to give a detailed account of how the law and nursing interact as this is a vast subject and there are already several excellent textbooks devoted to that theme. Nor will we look in detail at specialized areas of the law such as mental health or child care. What we shall be doing, however, is introducing a number of key legal principles which directly impact upon nurses seeking to expand their scope of practice and reviewing them in the light of the UKCC Scope document and the many changes in practice that are underway at present.

The nature of the law

'The law' is a very wide concept and it is essential to know something of the structure of the law and its origins before looking at particular areas that impact upon clinical practice. The law is broadly divided into two parts, civil and criminal law. The picture is further complicated by the fact that there are different legal systems in England (and Wales) and Scotland while the European courts have increasing amounts of influence on events in the UK due to our membership of the European Union. The law originates either by Act of Parliament (Statutes) or as a result of case law in which previous judgements and decisions influence subsequent cases as there is no formal Act of Parliament (common law). Generally speaking, in criminal law, offences are punishable by the state and usually involve law laid down by Acts of Parliament (Statutes) and the burden of proof involves the prosecution establishing their case 'beyond all reasonable doubt'. In civil law an individual is usually considered to have been wronged in such a way that he or she is entitled to compensation. Common law tends to dominate civil cases and the emphasis is on proving the case 'on the balance of probabilities' which is a lesser burden of proof. Such a civil wrong against a person is called a 'tort' in legal terminology.

Many minor criminal cases are dealt with in magistrates' courts and only the more serious offences go to trial by jury at the Crown Court. Even so, such cases have to be initially heard in a magistrates' court before committal to the more senior Crown Court. Sitting above the Crown Court are the High Courts of which the Queen's Bench Division deals with criminal cases. The next rung on the legal ladder is the Court of Appeal, consisting of senior judges known as Lord Justices of Appeal and, finally, above them are the Law Lords in the House of Lords. These final stages of the judicial system hear appeals against decisions made lower down the system and hand down definitive judgements on cases.

Civil cases involving damages of under £50 000 are normally dealt with by a judge sitting in the County Courts, although if the amounts claimed in damages are more substantial the case will go direct to the High Court where it will be heard in either the Chancery or Family Division (McHale et al., 1998). Appeals may go to the Court of Appeal and eventually the Law Lords as in criminal cases.

There are other types of court that the nurse may be involved in of which the coroner's court is perhaps the best known. Its function is to establish the cause of death of an individual, not to assign blame to any named person for that death. Nurses giving evidence in a coroner's court hearing into the death of a patient, however, often find it a very stressful and difficult experience as, despite what has been said in the previous sentence, there is often an element of implied blame, particularly involving the family of the deceased. Tribunals are less formal hearings at which a nurse may be required to give evidence or at which a nurse may bring a case such as for unfair dismissal in an industrial tribunal. Public enquiries may look into serious problems that have affected health care such as the Bristol Royal Infirmary cardiac surgery affair and, as such, have formal rules of evidence and often sit under the chairmanship of a judge.

Legal issues surrounding expansion of the nursing role are most likely to be brought up in civil courts and consequently this chapter will now focus on the civil law and the key areas of concern.

'Am I covered to do this?'

This common concern of many nurses makes a good starting point to explore what the civil law has to say. Key points to consider in answering this question are:

- ❏ What do we mean by covered?
- ❏ Covered against whom?
- ❏ Covered by whom?

To some nurses 'covered' may mean protection against being sued by a patient. However, every individual is liable for their actions in law and wearing a nursing uniform does not convey immunity from the due process of law. The nurse can never be protected in some way from being the subject of a patient complaint and possible legal action. The concept of accountability comes into play here for, as we shall see in the next chapter, the nurse is *individually* accountable for his or her actions at all times. Following the orders of a senior nurse or a doctor does not excuse the nurse, he or she is still accountable.

An alternative understanding of 'covered' is that the nurse is not personally liable for payment of damages to a patient. This is incorrect in theory as personal liability means just that, you are personally liable. However, in practice, the principle of vicarious liability means that the employer can be held liable for the actions of employees at all times unless that employee was acting for their own personal gain or undertaking work that they were not authorized to carry out. The general approach to such cases is that the plaintiff follows the principle of vicarious liability and usually brings the case against the employer rather than the individual nurse because, apart from anything else, they hope to recover a larger sum in damages that way (Young, 1994). Employers may, however, recover a contribution to the costs involved from employees, although there is NHS guidance that Trusts should not attempt to do this (NHS Executive, 1996).

In order therefore to be 'covered' by the principle of vicarious liability, the nurse has to ensure that he or she is working within boundaries that are approved by the employer. In expanding practice this therefore requires careful discussions with medical and other colleagues so that all parties know what the nurse is doing. This should be followed by obtaining a written statement defining how the nurse has expanded practice (preferably including any protocols that have been developed) which is signed by a senior manager of the Trust or the Practice Manager in the case of a Practice Nurse. This may sound rather bureaucratic but it is good practice to have all parties aware of the new role the nurse has developed and to have their written agreement. Should there be a problem with a patient subsequently, this is your insurance policy as the principle of vicarious liability can be clearly shown to apply as you were acting within your area of authority, as agreed by your employer. The other lesson to be learnt from this discussion concerns the temptation to do unofficial favours for people that do not form part of your contracted work. This temptation should be resisted as you are acting outside your contract and, it could be argued, you might even be doing so for personal gain.

The A&E nurse for example who feels something really should be done to meet the health needs of the homeless and who sets up an unofficial clinic at a local hostel could not claim vicarious liability if something went wrong. He or she would be in even more trouble if she had been using NHS equipment to run her unofficial clinic as this might be construed as theft. Mental health nurses carrying out outreach work in the community or nurse practitioners developing services for marginalized groups in society, such as prostitutes or drug users, should also think carefully about establishing vicarious liability for the same reasons. They should ensure there is no question of personal gain, they are operating within their contract of employment and that their employer knows and approves of what they are doing. Only in that way can they avoid placing themselves in a very exposed position beyond the protection offered to employees by vicarious liability.

Even if you have ensured that you comply with the principles of vicarious liability, there is still the possibility of the patient choosing to sue you personally despite the advice of their solicitor to sue your employer. Perhaps the motive for such an action would be revenge rather than recovering the maximum amount of money as compensation for the wrong suffered.

To return to the original point about being 'covered', meaning 'insured', the key issues are that you must be aware of the principles of vicarious liability and observe them at all times but, as a back up, arrange your own indemnity insurance in the eventuality that you find yourself being sued personally or your employer chooses to disregard NHS guidelines and tries to recover damages from you personally. Membership of the Royal College of Nursing or a similar body automatically gives the nurse full indemnity insurance cover against such eventualities. However, if you are going to pioneer some radical new area of practice development, it would be wise to check with the RCN that their policy would include protection for your new role.

Answering the question 'covered against whom?' leads into a discussion about accountability, which will be explored in depth in the next chapter. Suffice it to say that not only the patient (or their family) may take action against you, so may the UKCC if professional misconduct is suggested and so may your employer. It is wise therefore in developing new roles to remember that you may be called before the UKCC or your employer to justify your practice. Consult documents such as the *Code of Professional Conduct* and the *Scope of Professional Practice* to ensure that you are acting in a way that is consistent with UKCC requirements and also consult your job description and contract of employment. If substantial changes are being made to your practice, you should seek a new contract and job description to reflect your new role in order that there can be no ambiguity or dispute at a later date as to what you should or should not be doing. RCN members would do well to consult the RCN about new roles and the possibility of renegotiating contracts and job descriptions. Members of other unions should contact local officials of their union for advice in the same way.

The above discussion should have answered the third question of 'covered by whom?' As long as you are acting within your job description and not for personal gain the principle of vicarious liability applies and any damages involved should be paid by your employer. It is as well, however, to adopt a belt and braces approach and arrange your own indemnity insurance through membership of the RCN or other equivalent body. It would be very naive, and unprofessional, to rely on verbal reassurances from medical colleagues to the effect, 'Don't worry, I'll cover you for that'. That approach only reinforces the subservience of nursing to medicine and undermines the case for increasing degrees of autonomy and practice development. Good teamwork requires that medical colleagues know what we are doing and are in agreement with our practice, however nurses can make their *own* provision in the event of problems or patient complaints.

Expanding practice and the problem of negligence

Fear of legal action undoubtedly looms large in the minds of many nurses when considering taking on new roles. A good understanding of what the law expects from nurses is therefore essential if nurses are to expand practice confidently and safely. The problem is that, as civil law tends to be judge made and is therefore based on previous cases, some of which may have occurred decades ago long before expansion of nursing roles was an issue, the rulings involved tend to be about doctors and we have to translate them into a nursing context. There is therefore a fundamental assumption that the legal principles involved in medical rulings can be applied to nurses. Taking this assumption on board, we can now turn our attention to the legal definition of negligence which, cited by Young (1994) is as follows:

> Negligence is the omission to do something which a reasonable man, guided upon these considerations which ordinarily regulate the conduct of human affairs, would do, or to do something which a prudent and reasonable man would not do.

> Blyth v Birmingham Water Works 1891
> Cited in Young (1994) p.27.

The sexist language of the Victorian era can be brought up to date by replacing the word 'man' with 'nurse' and then you have a clear definition which has stood the test of time. There are two very important points in this definition, the first of which is that an omission to do something can be just as negligent as doing something unwise or wrong. Doing nothing in a difficult situation is therefore not an option for the nurse as that is just as negligent as doing the wrong thing. The other key point is the cautious language used, words such as 'ordinary', 'prudent' and 'reasonable', suggest that the law is not looking for outstanding excellence but rather an average, competent, safe pair of hands. There is much debate surrounding what is reasonable of course. The argument hinges on the question, reasonable by whose standards? Would a specialist nurse operating with a high degree of autonomy in an area such as breast care or bereavement counselling be expected to perform only at the standard of a recently qualified D grade staff nurse on a general ward? If a nurse expands his or her role as a nurse practitioner and is seeing patients with undifferentiated health problems and acting with a high degree of autonomy, should he or she be as competent as a recently appointed practice nurse who might have had a career break of several years for family reasons or crucially, should he or she be working at the same standard as a GP? These questions will be returned to shortly but first we have to see how the law develops this basic concept of negligence further.

In order to win damages for negligence the person bringing the case (plaintiff in England, pursuer in Scotland) must establish their case against the following three tests:

❏ The defendant owed the plaintiff a duty of care
❏ There was a breach in that duty of care
❏ The breach in the duty of care led to harm which was not too distant in time from the original incident and was reasonably foreseeable.

The nurse obviously owes the patient a duty of care while on duty. A situation which causes much debate is what happens when the nurse is off duty and witnesses an accident or a person suddenly taken ill. Views on this subject are divided among legal experts. Dimond (1993) states that 'There is no duty in law to volunteer help', and McHale *et al.* (1998 p.17) consider it unlikely that the courts would find there was 'an express legal duty to rescue a stranger'. However, Young (1994) states that the law does not accept an off-duty nurse has no duty of care. Apart from accountability in law, the nurse is also accountable to the UKCC and Castledine (1993) has described a case in which an off-duty nurse who refused to render first aid was reported to the UKCC and found guilty of professional misconduct, although not removed from the Register. The nurse is also accountable to her fellow nurses, herself and her own conscience. The refusal to assist is a poor advertisement for an occupation that prides itself upon the title 'The Caring Profession' and such a nurse would be badly letting down all her colleagues. Finally, could that nurse sleep with herself at night knowing she did nothing to help? Off-duty nurses in Omagh on that dreadful day in August 1998 had no hesitation in rendering first aid among the carnage left by the terrorist bombing, even when some of them were badly injured themselves. Let any nurse who would walk on past the scene of an accident remember the example set by the nurses of Omagh.

The second test in a negligence case means that the onus is on the plaintiff to prove that there has been a breach in the duty of care that is consistent with the basic philosophy that a person is innocent until proven guilty. Such proof requires legal assistance and, consequently, in the past individuals have usually required legal aid to help them meet the costs of pursuing a case. Escalating legal aid costs (which have to be met by the tax payer) have led the government to try to remove damages cases from legal aid and instead introduce the so-called 'no win no fee' system whereby solicitors are only paid a fee if they win the case. The likely impact of this change is that fewer cases will go to court as solicitors will only pursue cases they are confident of winning, while other dispute resolution strategies will become more important such as the growing Alternative Dispute Resolution (ADR) approach (Jarvis, 1998). While there is some concern that these changes may deny patients access to justice, it also has to be remembered that many cases only come to court as a last resort as the family cannot find out what actually went wrong. If the NHS was prepared to be more open and honest with patients, turning the rhetoric of 'patients as partners' into reality, there might be less litigation anyway.

The final point about harm occurring is crucial as if no actual harm occurs as a result of the negligence, the plaintiff cannot win their case however incompetent the nurse may have been. That does not of course remove the nurse's accountability to their employer and to the UKCC either of whom may take action, depending upon the nature of the case. Young (1994) cites an interesting case *(Barnett v. Chelsea and Kensington HMC 1969)* which illustrates the importance of this point. A patient had accidentally and unknowingly ingested poison and presented at the accident and emergency department in the small hours of the morning complaining of abdominal pain. The doctor on duty refused to come and see the man who died shortly afterwards. Clearly the doctor owed a duty of care and that duty of care was breached, however, the court ruled that as the man had ingested a fatal dose of poison that was untreatable, no harm occurred as a result of the breach in the duty of care as he would have died anyway. The case therefore failed. At the opposite end of the scale, if the nurse made a drug error that had no harmful effect on the patient such as giving 10 mg of diazepam instead of 5 mg, this too would not constitute a case for negligence.

Nurses working in A&E, especially in expanded roles such as nurse practitioners and triage nurses, must be acutely aware of the duty of care they owe a patient. There is a commonly held view that many A&E patients are 'inappropriate attenders'; a concept which has been criticized by many, including Walsh (1996) whose research demonstrated that it is not the patient who is inappropriate but often the service offered. Whatever feelings a nurse may have about the patient who presents at A&E with a condition that is neither an accident nor an emergency, that nurse owes a duty of care to the patient which will be breached by simply telling the patient to go away or ignoring them in the hope that they will get fed up of waiting and leave. However, if the nurse practitioner assesses the patient and then refers him/her to another agency (e.g. GP) without offering treatment, and that referral will not be detrimental to the outcome of the patient's condition, that could be argued to be fulfilling the department's duty of care and would be a safer course of action to adopt. In order to ensure that nurses are operating within the principle of vicarious liability, the department should have agreement from the Trust that nurse practitioners are allowed to make such decisions. Patients who refuse to cooperate with treatment in A&E after the nurse has explained fully what the consequences are, can be allowed to leave without fear of breaching the duty of care principle as it is their choice to refuse treatment. Needless to say such refusal should be carefully documented.

The phrase 'reasonably foreseeable' is very important in the third test for negligence. If the patient's notes have written on them in large red letters 'Allergic to iodine' and the nurse decides to treat a wound with a dressing containing iodine, then an allergic reaction and harm are foreseeable consequences of her actions. However, if the patient is not known to be allergic to iodine *and, if the nurse has checked for allergies in her assessment,* then any subsequent reaction could not be seen as reasonably foreseeable and therefore the nurse's actions are not negligent. This raises the issues of a more thorough assessment and history taking process than has normally been the case in nursing and also the importance of documentation. As nurses work in increasingly autonomous ways, moving away from the sheltered waters of medical protection, they have to learn new assessment techniques in order to practise safely.

The issue of timing is also important as an adult may bring an action for negligence up to 3 years after the incident while in the case of a child, the action can be brought any time up to the child's 21st birthday. This long time delay means it is essential that the nurse has good quality documentation about all patients, as apart from anything else, the frailties of human memory are such that he or she would be unlikely to remember very much with any degree of accuracy and confidence. If there is any doubt in court as to what actually happened, the plaintiff is usually given the benefit of that doubt, hence the importance of accurate records which not only note what happened, but also *what did not happen.* Sometimes, recording a negative is just as important as recording what did happen. It is essential that the plaintiff establishes harm occurred directly as a result of the nurse's negligence rather than arguing that the nurse's negligence was one of several possible causes, which again underlines the importance of clear documentation.

The increasingly autonomous roles which nurses are now developing must be matched by improvements in documentation which go far beyond the traditional nursing process care plan which is often of very poor quality. There is a strong case for a single multidisciplinary patient document that all staff can use. The increasing use of critical pathways facilitates accurate, multidisciplinary documentation and also has the advantage of providing an evidence-based plan of care to which the patient has access. This makes it easier to defend any subsequent legal action as the Trust can argue from a position of strength that the care planned was provided according to the document, and that the care was 'best practice', as the pathway was drawn up by the multidisciplinary team based on the best evidence available at the time.

The definition of negligence cited above hinges upon the key word 'reasonable' and it is to a case in 1957 that we have to look for a legal definition *(Bolam v Friern HMC)* of this term. The judgement in this case has become well known as the Bolam test and Mr Justice McNair, the judge in this case, defined it as follows:

> The test is the standard of the ordinary skilled man exercising and professing to have that specialist skill. A man need not possess the highest expert skill; it is well established law that it is sufficient if he exercises the ordinary skill of an ordinary competent man exercising that particular art.
>
> Cited in McHale et al. (1998 p.19)

Once again we substitute the word 'nurse' for 'man' to arrive at a working translation for nursing practice. A key section of the judgement in this case stated that as long as there was a responsible body of opinion of the view that whatever had been done was correct, then it did not constitute negligence even if there was an equally strong opposing view. The implications of this ruling have been summarized by Pennels (1997a) as follows:

❏ The standard of care required is that which would be considered acceptable and current practice *at the time*. This rules out claims that may be brought with the benefit of hindsight if evidence subsequently suggests that what was done at the time was perhaps not for the best. It also highlights the need for the nurse to keep up to date with new evidence and changing practice guidelines.
❏ An ordinary level of nursing skill and competence is sufficient while the highest standards possible are not necessary in a strict legal sense.
❏ Nurses must follow standards and guidelines laid down by professional, local and national bodies.
❏ If you possess specialist skills you must also exercise the ordinary skills of the RN.

So long as the nurse practises in a mainstream fashion, with the support of a responsible body of nursing opinion, then he or she is on safe ground even if other nurses disagree. The nurse, however, who is exploiting the *Scope of Professional Practice* guidelines to push back the boundaries of practice may find herself working in an area where there is not a 'responsible body of nursing opinion'. Pioneers rarely have that luxury and, almost by definition, will be blazing the trail for others to follow. This therefore leaves the specialist nurse or the nursing pioneer still looking for a definition of 'reasonable' to help her guide practice.

The growth of the evidence-based practice movement may lead to this accepted legal wisdom being challenged. Expert opinion is regarded as the weakest form of evidence behind evidence-based national clinical guidelines, systematic reviews and individual reviews of the published evidence (Morgan, 1997). It should only be resorted to in the absence of research-based evidence. Authorities such as Cullum and DiCenso (1998) point out there are many examples of healthcare interventions which anecdotally have been claimed to be successful, but which have failed the test of randomized controlled trials. This leads these authors strongly to disagree with the assertion that individual clinical experience is a better source of evidence than research-based evidence. The implications for the nurse involved in practice expansion are that he or she should, at all times, ensure practice is evidence based and can be justified in the literature while, in the not too distant future, the validity of the Bolam Test may well be under serious pressure in the Courts.

A firm evidence base for practice helps us to decide what to do, but still leaves the question of how to do it and to what standards, open for debate. We have to return to the question of reasonable by whose standards? Standards depend, among other things, on experience and expertise and the view of the law is that the inexperience of an individual clinician can never be a defence against a claim for negligence. This was well summarized by Mr Justice Glidewell (Wilsher v Essex AHA 1986 cited by Pennels, 1997a) who stated that trainee doctors must be judged by the same standards as their more experienced colleagues otherwise inexperience would frequently be used as a defence against negligence claims (Pennels, 1997a). The standard that should be achieved is that which the *post requires* not that of the individual clinician. This means that what matters are the skills needed to perform the job safely and competently, not the skills the nurse can offer (Pennels, 1997a). If the nurse does not have the skills and underpinning knowledge to perform a task safely then she simply should not be doing it. This point is particularly pertinent given the plethora of nurse practitioners who have been appointed in the last few years, many of whom have had only a limited amount of in-service training to equip them for their new role, rather than a rigorous course such as the RCNI BSc Nurse Practititioner course. Kloss (1988) has summarized the arguments by pointing out that a nurse undertaking a task for which she has had insufficient training may well be judged negligent, even if acting on the orders of a doctor. Kloss goes on to reiterate that if the nurse takes on a role which was once thought medical, she will be judged by the standards of a reasonable doctor.

The nurse practitioner seeing patients with undifferentiated health problems in primary care therefore should be judged by the standards of a GP, while her counterpart in A&E should be expected to achieve the standard of an SHO as this is what the *post* requires. The nurse specialist developing increasingly autonomous practice in managing a case load in outpatients would also be expected to achieve a similar medical standard of competence as that is what the post requires. The nurse therefore has to combine bringing advanced and traditional nursing skills to the new role with the standards expected of a competent doctor where relevant to the post. This reinforces the point already made about assessment and the need for taking a structured medical history and carrying out a focused physical examination to the standard of a medical practitioner if the nurse is working in a largely autonomous role, undertaking practice, of which some was previously the province of medicine. This is not an unreasonable position when viewed from the patients' perspective.

A term that is often used in conjunction with negligence is liability, which simply means that a person is responsible for the outcome of their actions. A nurse is therefore liable to the patient through the civil law, the UKCC via the *Code of Professional Conduct* and the employer as a result of the contract of employment. Liability to the patient is usually discharged via the employer under the principle of vicarious liability (see p.69) and it is the employer who is usually sued for damages in the event of negligence being proved. Pennels (1997b) points out that the degree of liability (and hence damages) can be reduced if it can be shown that the patient was partially responsible for the harm that occurred (for example, they failed to follow instructions) or if the nurse's negligent act is not the sole cause of harm or was only a contributory factor. Employers defending a claim may therefore be very keen to establish that any of the above situations is true in order to reduce the amount of damages that have to be paid.

The following summary lists simple steps that can provide protection against liability for negligence:

- ❏ Be sure of your personal competence and think carefully about the skills required of the post rather than the skills you already have
- ❏ Ensure there is a strong evidence base for your practice
- ❏ Document all care thoroughly, including things that have not happened as well as things that have
- ❏ Take all complaints seriously and act promptly in line with local policies for complaint resolution
- ❏ Ensure your employer knows what you are doing in your clinical practice and that it is within your contract of employment
- ❏ Check your professional indemnity insurance if there is a significant change in your practice.

The problem of consent

As the nurse becomes increasingly autonomous in his or her scope of practice, the issue of consent must be borne in mind. The requirement for consent has both a legal and an ethical origin. Ethically it is clearly wrong to do things to patients without their consent and the Code of Conduct makes this clear. However, it also requires us to always act in the patient's best interests, which can lead to debate as to whether some actions are always in the patient's best interests. The nurse who sees an alcoholic patient drinking alcohol for example, might consider it in his best interests not to have that drink, but does that give the nurse the right to remove the bottle from the patient against his wishes? There are times when the Code of Conduct contains such inherent contradictions and the nurse has to try to negotiate a solution. Apart from being aware of Trust policy and guidelines for dealing with such situations, he or she should also be aware of how the law stands on such matters, for as ever there is the burden of triple accountability to contend with, i.e. accountability to the employer, the UKCC and in law.

The area of the civil law that largely governs this area is the law of trespass. Most of us are familiar with trespass as a concept that applies to property, however, it also applies to the person. In civil law, as opposed to the criminal law, any attempt or threat of applying unlawful force to the person is an assault for which he may claim compensation. No physical contact needs to occur for the patient to claim assault under civil law, all that matters is that the action is unlawful, i.e. without the consent of the patient. The term battery is used when actual contact with the patient is made and, unlike negligence, the patient does not have to prove any harm occurred to pursue a claim for damages. If the patient gives consent to an action or procedure there is no case to answer for assault or battery and, if the contact made was accidental, again there is no case (although there might be a question of negligence!).

Consent can either be in writing, verbal or implied. The patient rolling up his sleeve as the nurse approaches holding a sphygmomanometer is giving implied consent to having his blood pressure checked. No words are spoken but the actions of the patient are consent. The nurse must of course have still explained what is happening, the patient rolling his sleeve up in anticipation of having his blood pressure checked is not giving consent to the nurse sticking a needle in his vein and withdrawing blood. Dimond (1995) points out two potentially dangerous assumptions that may be made about implied consent. The fact that the patient is in hospital or at the health centre does not mean they have consented 'by implication' to whatever the staff wish to do, actions still have to be explained and permission obtained. The second assumption concerns the patient who is unconscious. Lack of awareness or the ability to communicate does not give staff implied consent, however critical the situation. You must remember that what is happening is that care is being given, *without consent,* in light of his serious condition, in response to the duty of care that the hospital has to the individual. Any subsequent legal action would be defended from the point of view of the duty of care, not implied consent.

Verbal consent is given whenever the patient states that they agree to a procedure and is usually regarded as sufficient in many situations, taking blood for example. There is always the difficulty in any subsequent dispute that there is no written record of consent and a case may become little more than the word of the nurse against the word of the patient. It is worth noting that in the example above, taking blood, the assumption is always that any tests performed will be in the patient's best interests, therefore, *any* test which meets that criterion may be performed. This is the legal basis for screening for conditions such as AIDS and possibly in the future, BSE, even though the patient was not told at the time that their blood would be so tested.

The opposite of verbal consent is refusal to cooperate with treatment and possibly self-discharge. If the patient refuses to allow treatment then, apart from the very special circumstances of being detained under the appropriate section of the Mental Health Act (MHA) which permits treatment, no treatment can occur. If the patient decides to walk out of the hospital, despite attempts at reasonable persuasion and explanations of the possible consequences of such actions, he has to be allowed to walk. He cannot be restrained. Careful documentation of the facts is of course essential. It should be remembered that Section 4 of the MHA, while permitting emergency admission for 72 hours, only permits assessment, not treatment. Treatment is permitted under Section 3 which initially runs for 6 months.

The discussion about verbal consent opens up the debate about informed consent, which is particularly acute when consent is required in writing. This should always be obtained for any procedure involving a significant element of risk, such as surgery. Nurses expanding their roles in areas such as preoperative assessment of patients should not, however, become involved in obtaining written consent for a procedure to be undertaken by a doctor. If the procedure varies at all from that to which the patient consented, then there is a case for legal action. Nurses often have reservations about how informed is the consent that many patients give when they sign consent forms after a brief explanation by a doctor. However, the solution is not for the nurse to undertake the consenting, but rather to discharge his or her duty of care to the patient by informing the doctor that the patient has not fully understood, is having second thoughts or would like to discuss the operation further. Such action should be carefully documented in the nursing notes for future reference.

The nub of this issue is the thorny question of whether the patient knew enough for the consent to be valid, i.e. informed consent. The patient may bring an action for negligence if they felt they had not been given sufficient information to make a valid decision about consent. Harm must therefore have ensued (see p. 72). This raises the key question of what constitutes informed consent or, put another way, how much should the patient be told about the possible side effects of treatment? Dimond (1995) has summarized the current legal position as indicating that the patient should only be told as much as the doctor thinks he needs to know to make a decision. The nurse in such a situation therefore should follow the same principle to stay within legal boundaries. There is no legal requirement to tell the patient every possible side effect or risk involved in a procedure. The Bolam test (p. 75) is cited here for, as long as there is a body of opinion which supports the view that a patient should be told about complication X but not side effect Y, then that is sufficient to withhold telling the patient about Y. Even if the patient asks a specific question about a specific complication, rather than a general question about possible side effects, the doctor (and hence nurse) is under no legal obligation to respond. An alternative legal view holds that, as the doctor is entitled to withhold information, then there can be no breach in the duty of care if such information is withheld. The effect is the same, the patient may be unable to win a claim for negligence even if information about side effects has been withheld.

The nurse wrestling with the UKCC Code of Conduct, which requires truth telling and acting in the best interests of the patient at all times, may find this legal view problematical. Taylor (1999) points out that the principle of utility, i.e. there may be times when, from a pragmatic point of view, the professional judgement that some information should be withheld is not morally unacceptable. This can only follow after a careful consideration of the benefits and harm that might ensue from disclosing less than 100% of what is known. There may indeed be times when withholding information is in the patient's best interests. Perhaps nursing needs a debate about the issue of telling the patient the truth at all times, including listing every possible known side effect for every treatment, the results of which may be to scare a patient off a treatment for a one in a million risk. A more sophisticated approach to risk assessment is needed than that which has characterized nursing practice in the past. A one in a million risk of an adverse side effect if a treatment is given has to be weighed against the implications of not giving the treatment. It is as well therefore to rehearse the arguments in advance with your employers and medical colleagues, as well as nurse manager so that there is an agreed set of local guidelines to follow. Expert opinion from bodies such as the RCN or UKCC could also be obtained in order that the nurse moving into increasingly autonomous areas of practice may avoid becoming entangled in the sometimes contradictory web of accountability issues and informed consent.

One other key area of the law on consent which must be addressed concerns children. Paediatric nurses are usually well aware of the differing legal position of children, however, nurses in other areas such as A&E, Practice Nurses and Primary Health Care Nurse Practitioners also need to be equally aware. Although the age of majority is 18, young persons of 16 and 17 can give full consent to medical treatment. However, their parents can also give consent. When the views of both parties agree there is no problem, but a potential problem can occur when their respective opinions diverge as the law can be interpreted to mean that the young person can give consent at the same time as the parent refuses it, or vice versa. In such a situation a legal decision would be considered in the light of the individual circumstances and could support either the patient or the parent's position, possibly leaving the nurse or doctor in the wrong. Once again this emphasizes the need for the careful drawing up of guidelines in advance of situations.

When the young person is aged under 16, normally the parents' consent is required for any treatment. However, there are exceptions, the most famous of which has become known as 'Gillick competency', so called because of the case which established circumstances in which a minor aged under 16 could be treated without parental consent. The case revolved around a prescription for oral contraceptives given by a doctor to a girl aged under 16. The girl's mother (Mrs Gillick) objected and the case finally ended up being decided by the House of Lords.

Their ruling was that the girl could receive contraception without her parents' consent providing she was mature enough to understand fully the advice given; she was likely to have sexual intercourse anyway; she could not be persuaded to change her mind; and unless she received contraceptive advice or treatment her health would suffer and therefore it was in her best interests to receive the treatment (Dimond, 1995). This judgement has created the concept of Gillick competency and has implications far beyond contraception. It has opened the door for young persons under 16 to receive treatment and advice in exceptional circumstances, without parental consent. However, the nurse should tread very carefully and try to involve the parents at all times in dealing with a patient under 16 who presents alone for treatment.

Emergency treatment of a child without parental consent follows the same principle as treating an adult. There is a clear duty of care to the patient and staff must act in the patient's best interests. In an emergency situation, the defence of acting to save life would always cover staff against any subsequent claim for damages due to trespass upon the person.

The issue of informed consent has been discussed earlier and the dilemma highlighted as to whether patients should be told everything or given only the information which the doctor thinks is sufficient to make a decision. In the case of seriously injured or very sick children, the breaking of such bad news to parents may leave them so numbed and shocked that it is impossible for them to make a considered choice about treatment (Taylor, 1999). As a result, the expertise and support of medical and nursing staff is essential in helping parents come to terms with the devastating news that their child is unconscious after a serious head injury or has been diagnosed as having a disease such as leukaemia. As Taylor points out, in these situations, parents want experts acting in what they consider to be their child's best interests, which is not the same as somebody telling them every single possible complication and potential problem and, as a result, expecting them to make near impossible decisions about their child's treatment.

There may be situations which, at that moment, are not a life or death emergency but where treatment is deemed necessary, yet the parents withhold consent. The Children Act allows for the health authority to apply to make the child a ward of court, this effectively removes the parents' legal right to object to treatment. Alternatively an application may be made for a 'prohibited steps order' under the Children Act which stops the parent exercising parental responsibility without the consent of the court. A further provision in the act allows for a 'specific issue order', whereby the court rules on a specific question of medical treatment (McHale *et al.*, 1998). Senior Trust management must be involved at an early stage if any of the steps mentioned in this paragraph is likely to be needed.

The whole area of child protection lies outside the scope of this text. Any nurse working with children has a professional responsibility, however, to ensure he or she is fully aware of local policies in this crucial area and knows when and how to contact the appropriate agencies such as social services, police and health visitors.

Prescription of medicines

The legal position of nurses with regard to prescribing powers has been the subject of much debate throughout the 1990s. The Medicinal Products (Prescription by Nurses) Act of 1992 was a piece of primary legislation that was achieved after much intensive lobbying by the RCN and other nursing groups. It opened the door to nurses having prescribing rights, although its implementation has been slow and frustrating. Only now are limited prescribing rights (from a very slim nurses' formulary) being rolled out across the UK to nurses in possession of Health Visiting and District Nursing qualifications after many years of trials and pilot studies. Meanwhile, a major report (the Crown Report, 1999) is proposing radical changes which will completely overtake the limited changes being introduced as a result of allowing community nurse prescribing from the nurses' formulary to go ahead.

There are actually three legal definitions of the term prescribing which the nurse needs to be aware of and which are quoted in the Crown Report (1999) as follows:

❏ To order in writing the supply of a prescription only medicine (POM) for a named patient
❏ To authorize by means of an NHS prescription the supply of any medicine, not just a prescription only medicine (POM), at public expense
❏ To advise a patient on suitable care or medication, including medicine which may be purchased over the counter. This latter definition is only used occasionally.

This should be differentiated from the term supply, which means to provide a medicine directly to a patient or carer for administration. Pharmacists are the normal route of supply for POMs but doctors and dentists may also supply medicines to patients or they can direct nurses or other health professionals to supply medicines in hospitals or health centres. The term administration simply means to give a medicine either by introduction into the body by any route or by application to the surface of the body. A written prescription is required only for POMs and doctors and dentists have been the only people legally able to write out such prescriptions for human use. The other two categories of medicines besides POMs are pharmacy (P) and general sales list (GSL) medicines. Pharmacy drugs can only be sold or supplied by a pharmacist or under the direct supervision of a pharmacist on registered pharmacy premises, while GSL medications can be sold to the general public at any lockable business premises.

The rapid growth in the complexity of health care, changes in patient expectations, increased knowledge and skills of a range of non-medical practitioners and changes in interdisciplinary working practices, have all contributed to a momentum for change in the traditional patterns of drug prescribing. Group protocol schemes have been devised in recent years in order to meet the changing requirements of health care practice and to keep within the law. These schemes were reviewed in 1998 by a team led by Dr June Crown which found a wide range of practices. This review defined a group protocol as:

> A specific written instruction for the supply or administration of named medicines in an identified clinical situation.
> (Crown, 1998)

The protocol is drawn up locally by doctors and pharmacists and must be approved by the employer after consultation with appropriate professional bodies. It is used for groups rather than individually identified patients.

Crown (1998) states that they have been introduced to reduce patient waiting times, improve access to treatment, make better use of professional skills and maximize effective use of resources. However, in their review, the Crown team found that many group protocols did not measure up to the required standards for safe and effective practice. Reasons for this included lack of consultation with appropriate experts and professional bodies, muddled lines of accountability, imprecise clinical criteria or details about medicines involved and failure to take into account other existing guidelines. The Review Team therefore concluded that, while in the majority of cases medication should be provided on an individual basis, there was a place for group protocols, providing they were designed to improve patient care and took into account the issues raised above. Group protocols are therefore legal, providing they are correctly designed, unambiguous, have clear lines of accountability and precise clinical criteria built into them. Their role in health care delivery should, however, be limited and they may well be subsumed within a more radical reform of prescribing which is now being proposed.

The potential for confusion that can arise in the field of group protocols is highlighted by Pediani (1998). He argues that within the present legal framework, protocols could be written in such a way as to allow specialist pain control nurses to vary them depending upon the patient's condition, and for other nurses to follow the varied protocol. However, Pediani observes that many pain control specialist nurses would consider asking another nurse to administer medication under such circumstances as 'prescribing'. This is despite the fact that the only legal prescribing involved has already been carried out when the doctor wrote the original protocol and accepted responsibility for it. The pain specialist nurse would use his or her expertise to judge when the clinical conditions were such that another nurse could follow the protocol and in those circumstances could 'transcribe' the protocol onto the drug chart. The specialist nurse is therefore screening for the right conditions under which the protocol is activated.

An example quoted by Pediani concerns a patient on patient controlled analgesia (PCA) which is delivering morphine. A rash has developed causing local irritation. If the protocol allowed for the substitution of another opioid such as pethidine under such circumstances, the specialist nurse could delete the morphine prescription and replace it with pethidine, according to the overall protocol and then other nurses could follow the new analgesia regimen. This would bring immediate benefit to the patient and avoid lengthy delays while medical staff were brought to the ward to review the situation and rewrite the prescription.

Medical support for allowing specialist nurses to expand their practice in this way comes from Jones (1998), who reinforces the arguments that this will make for significant improvements in patient care, better use of skilled nursing time, closer monitoring of the patient's condition and more rapid adjustments of medication if needed and increased levels of autonomy for the nursing role. He also argues that specialist nurses acting in this way will be able to make a significant contribution to medical education about analgesia while improving overall teamwork between doctors and nurses. Trusts need to be bold and not be put off by the medico-legal confusion that surrounds this area as, if basic principles are adhered to, Jones and Pediani both argue safe and greatly improved practice can be developed for the patient. Such an approach is in line with the main thrust of clinical governance, which is about bringing decision making closer to the patient. Although there is legal opinion objecting to this approach and casting doubt over the competence of nurses in this field (Pennels, 1998), the last word belongs with Miaskowski (1998) writing from a North American perspective. She asks 'If the medical and nursing professions recognize the benefits of using protocols to manage acute post-operative pain, why is the legal system inhibiting this type of approach to a significant clinical problem?' As she observes the combination of quality imperatives and changes in junior medical staff mean that we can no longer carry on as we are and we have to find ways of bringing nursing expertise to bear on the problem of post-operative pain. Protocols are a major part of the answer to the problem until such time as the Crown Report (1999) is fully implemented.

The Crown Report of 1999 was an acknowledgement of the uncertainty that still surrounds prescribing and group protocols. It has made a series of radical recommendations to end the present *ad hoc* arrangements and place the prescribing and supply of medicines by others than doctors and dentists on a much firmer footing. The first major point is to invite new groups of professionals to apply for authority to prescribe in specific clinical areas. As the 1992 Prescription by Nurses Act was primary legislation, it may be that nurses already have such rights. Whatever the outcome of that debate, the next major point is that there should be two classes of new prescribers, independent and dependent prescribers. The former have responsibility for being the first point of contact and carrying out a thorough patient assessment before devising a plan of care, of which drug prescription may be a part. Nurse practitioners clearly fit within that description. Dependent precribers would have the power to vary prescriptions made by new independent prescribers and conventional medical staff, within an agreed treatment plan. There is much to read in the Crown Report and it may well be long after this book is published before there is final agreement and action on its recommendations. It is sincerely hoped that it will bring change to clarify the legal position of nurses involved in prescribing medication for patients, as the present situation is not in the interests of patients or nurses and is recognized by most doctors as needing urgent attention. In the interim, nurses working with group protocols should consult the 1998 Crown Report to ensure they are working in such a way as to be consistent with the recommendations for best practice that this report contains.

Summary

This chapter has discussed some of the key topics that impinge upon nurses expanding their scope of professional practice. We will finish where we began by reminding you of the importance of knowing key legal principles concerning issues such as negligence and consent together with the detail of your area of practice such as the Children or Mental Health acts. Increasing levels of autonomy and accountability make it axiomatic that nurses developing their roles understand what the law has to say about clinical practice. The right to expand practice will always be accompanied by increasing levels of responsibility, including responsibility within the law.

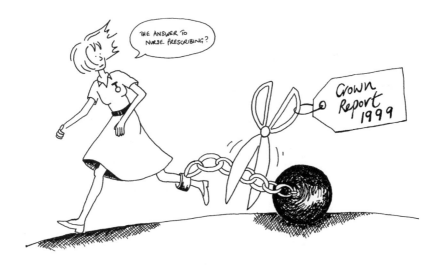

References

Castledine, G. (1993). Ethical implications of first aid. *British Journal of Nursing*, **2**, 4, 239–241.

Crown, J. (1998). *Review of Prescribing Supply and Administration of Medicines; A Report on the Supply and Administration of Medicines under Group Protocols.* London: DoH.

Crown, J. (1999). *Review of Prescribing, Supply and Administration of Medicines*. London: DoH.

Cullum, N. and DiCenso, A. (1998). Implementing evidence based nursing: some misconceptions. *Evidence Based Nursing*, **1**, 2, 38–40.

Dimond, B. (1993). Legal aspects of first aid and emergency care:2. *British Journal of Nursing*, **2**, 13, 692–694.

Dimond, B. (1995). *Legal Aspects of Nursing* (2nd edn). London: Prentice Hall.

Jarvis, J. (1998). Legal first aid. *Nursing Standard*, **12**, 49, 24.

Jones, M. (1998). Nurse prescribing in acute pain: The UK situation and the medical perspective. *Acute Pain*, **1**, 5, 44–46.

Kloss, D. (1988). Demarcation in medical practice; the extended role of the nurse. *Professional Negligence*, **4**, 2, 41–47.

Miaskowski, C. (1998). An idea whose time has come. *Acute Pain*, 5, 1, 5–6.

McHale, J., Tingle, J. and Peysner, J. (1998). *Law and Nursing*. Oxford: Butterworth-Heinemann.

Morgan, E. (1997). Clinical effectiveness. *Nursing Standard*, **11**, 34, 43–47.

NHS Executive (1996). *NHS Indemnity Arrangements for Clinical Negligence Claims in the NHS 96 HR 0024*. Leeds: DoH.

Pediani, R. (1998). Nurse prescribing in acute pain; the UK situation and the nursing perspective. *Acute Pain*, **1**, 5, 41–43.

Pennels, C. (1998). Nurse prescribing in acute pain; the UK situation and the legal perspective. *Acute Pain*, **5**, 1, 47–50.

Pennels, C. (1997a). Professional negligence. *Professional Nurse*, **13**, 1, 50–51.

Pennels, C. (1997b). Liability in negligence. *Professional Nurse*, **13**,1, 52–53.

Selden, J. (1689). Table Talk. In: 1892 edn of *Law*.

Taylor, B. (1999). Parental autonomy and consent to treatment. *Journal of Advanced Nursing*, **29**, 3, 570–576.

Taylor, B. (1999). Parental autonomy and consent to treatment. *Journal of Advanced Nursing*, **29**, 3. 570–576.

UKCC (1992). *The Scope of Professional Practice*. London: UKCC.

Walsh, M. (1996). *Accident and Emergency Nursing* (3rd edn). Oxford: Butterworth-Heinemann.

Young, A. (1994). *Law and Professional Conduct in Nursing*. London: Scutari.

is difficult to see how a nurse can be held accountable for something over which she has little or no authority. There is research evidence to support these views as Adamson *et al.* (1995) were able to show high levels of dissatisfaction among their sample of both UK and Australian hospital nurses, based upon perceptions of structural medical dominance and nursing's own lack of power and authority.

Any discussion of accountability must therefore recognize the problem of authority that faces nursing as a whole and the individual nurse in everyday practice. One of the key attributes of accountability is that it is very personal and individualistic. The rise of accountability in nursing came at the end of a period in British political history when the individual was paramount and society took second place. This Thatcherite creed of the 1980s spilled over into the 1990s when both the Scope document and the revised Code of Professional Conduct were being drafted by the UKCC. The linkage between the rise of accountability and the right wing political dogma of Thatcherism is probably not coincidental. When John Major took over from Mrs Thatcher as Prime Minister we were greeted with the named nurse initiative and the notion that every patient should have a nurse named as being responsible for their nursing care. This was a continuation of the same ideology. The named nurse initiative was compromised from the beginning by inadequate staffing levels; nurses' perceived lack of authority to act effectively on behalf of individual patients; lack of ownership of what was another top-down change; and a failure to explore fully what the concept meant, particularly in relation to associate nurses and the concept of primary nursing. These issues are reflected in the findings of Dooley (1999) whose small-scale study was handicapped by a poor response rate, but at least is one of the few attempts actually to research what nurses felt about the named nurse.

Accountability can make the contribution of each individual nurse visible. It is therefore necessary to have a clear view of what the goals are for each individual nurse and nursing team. Nurses cannot be held accountable unless there are unambiguous outcomes and standards against which performance can be measured. Clinical audit is therefore a key component of accountability, especially when linked to critical pathways or as Duff (1995) suggests the dynamic standard setting system (DySSSy). The DySSSy approach emphasizes the importance of nurses setting their own standards for care utilizing the familiar framework of structure, process and outcome. Criteria can then be derived to reflect these standards. The criteria are audited to measure progress towards achieving the agreed standards. Duff argues that as DySSSy allows nurses to set their own standards for nursing care which they can audit, it allows nursing to practice self-regulation and hence accountability. However, the real world of health care does not fall into neat compartments, one of which can be labelled 'nursing'. Health care is a complicated business with many practitioners all influencing patient care. This poses the question of how much care can be isolated for which nurses can be held solely accountable? It also links with the question of authority, for if nurses lack authority, can they be held accountable for failing to achieve certain goals?

There are further complications that Duff (1995) points out. She states that there are two approaches to quality assurance (QA); the traditional

Accountability

'To such a pitch of folly I am brought,
Being caught between the pull
Of the dark moon and the full'

W.B. Yeats, (1921)
The Double Vision of Michael Robartes

Introduction

During the 1990s, accountability became a much used word in the nursing literature. This poses the question whether this is merely a *'fin de siècle'* phenomenon that will fade with the passing century or whether nursing really has embraced accountability as a key professional concept. The problem with accountability is that the nurse finds him- or herself accountable to several different bodies at once. The result is that he or she is pulled in different directions by conflicting and opposing forces. To talk of the UKCC, the patient and your employer might not sound as sweet on the ear as the poetry of Yeats quoted above, but the sentiment is the same. Indeed, perhaps it is folly to try to hold nurses accountable in so many different ways when they have so little authority. Any discussion of accountability cannot ignore the twin issues of autonomy and authority. This linkage will be discussed in exploring the ramifications of expanding nursing practice and accountability. Despite being used in everyday conversation interchangeably with the word 'responsibility', accountability means something very different and the two words should not be confused. This chapter will therefore address the issue of differentiating between accountability and responsibility.

Accountability and responsibility

The various nursing bodies, tutors and ordinary nurses used to talk a great deal about the responsibilities of being a nurse. It was not the sort of occupation for people lacking a sense of responsibility and duty.

Responsibility means that the nurse is given a charge for which she is answerable. In other words you are given a job or a duty to perform which you are expected to carry out to the best of your ability. There was an implicit assumption that if the nurse did not know how, she would say so rather than carry on and place the patient at hazard. A moment's reflection suggests that nurses have to be responsible in this way and responsibility is therefore a necessary quality for any nurse. The problem comes when it is also seen as a sufficient quality, which was the case from Nightingale's time onwards. Responsibility and a sense of duty chimed nicely with the Victorian order of things when everybody knew their place, which, in the case of women, was doing what they were told, without demur. It is therefore a passive concept in which the nurse waits to be told what to do by either a senior nurse or a doctor.

This historical perspective on the problem of accountability and responsibility has been developed by McCann (1995). She points out that the bruising battle within nursing to establish registration, which culminated in the Nursing Registration Acts of 1919, led to a piece of legislation which divided nursing by setting up supplementary registers (e.g. male nurses, mental nurses, nurses of mental defectives etc.) and left all the decisions of the newly established General Nursing Council (GNC) subject to approval by the Minister of Health and both Houses of Parliament. Nursing was divided and had little absolute control over its affairs with the result that early efforts by the GNC to raise educational standards were thwarted by government interference as it was thought educational standards were being set too high and it would cost too much money. *Plus ça change, plus la même chose* as the French would say! The resulting apprenticeship system of training with its emphasis on obedience and following orders, rather than original thought, led to the growth of responsibility and duty as the main principles guiding nursing practice. As a result of the way nursing was established in the early years of the 20th century, nursing has had no legal status compared to medicine, no professional autonomy, a top heavy system of hierarchy within which the buck could always be passed to somebody else, and a system of apprenticeship training which frowned upon original thinking (McCann, 1995). It is little wonder therefore that duty and responsibility were all and accountability remained an alien concept until very recently.

Accountability was first introduced to nursing as a major theme in the 1992 version of the *UKCC Code of Professional Conduct* and the *Scope of Professional Practice* (UKCC, 1992). There are various definitions of the concept and perhaps the easiest way is think of the word from which accountability is derived, i.e. 'account'. Put simply, accountability means being able to give an account of your actions, to explain and justify why you did what you did. Jones (1996) sees it as encompassing responsibility for one's own actions and also being answerable for them. Rumsey (1997) expands on this simple concept by explaining that accountability involves:

❑ Assessing what is in the best interests of patients in sometimes complex situations

❑ Using nursing knowledge and your own judgemer upon a course of action
❑ Being able to explain and, if necessary, defend your action.

Accountability therefore involves responsibility, knowledge an able to justify your actions. It also involves the ability to make de and carry them through into practice, i.e. autonomy and authority. therefore a complex concept and one which would have been unthinka until recently given what we know of nursing history (McCann, 199! The issue of authority has, however, not been emphasized by the UKC(in their work on accountability and Hancock (1997) points out this glaring omission from documents such as Scope and the Code of Conduct. Hancock develops the argument further as she considers that at present there are areas where nurses cannot be held accountable as they are not involved in the decision making process. She cites the example of decisions concerning a patient's resuscitation status; this is still made usually by the medical staff without nursing input. The UKCC's brave words about accountability will count for nothing if institutions remain locked into fragmented and ritualistic approaches to practice, traditional power structures and controlling hierarchies (Hancock, 1997).

Accountability means that nurses:

❑ Are responsible for their actions at all times
❑ Can justify and explain their actions
❑ Have the authority to act in the way that they think is best for the patient.

Accountability, authority and autonomous practice

Hancock's criticism is well directed as authority lies at the heart of any debate about accountability. Nursing's subservient role within the NHS has been analysed by Ford and Walsh (1994) who drew upon the writings of both feminists and critical social theorists to argue that nursing constitutes an oppressed group with relatively little power and hence authority. Subsequent work by Parker (1995) continues the theme as sh argues that the relationships and structures which govern the distributic of power within hospitals only emphasize the disempowerment nursing which becomes invisible as a result. It is the privileged status medical power and knowledge that is the dominant force within he care, leaving nursing lacking in power and recognition. This challenges the UKCC's assertion that nurses are always accountable

Accountability

'To such a pitch of folly I am brought,
Being caught between the pull
Of the dark moon and the full'

W.B. Yeats, (1921)
The Double Vision of Michael Robartes

Introduction

During the 1990s, accountability became a much used word in the nursing literature. This poses the question whether this is merely a *'fin de siècle'* phenomenon that will fade with the passing century or whether nursing really has embraced accountability as a key professional concept. The problem with accountability is that the nurse finds him- or herself accountable to several different bodies at once. The result is that he or she is pulled in different directions by conflicting and opposing forces. To talk of the UKCC, the patient and your employer might not sound as sweet on the ear as the poetry of Yeats quoted above, but the sentiment is the same. Indeed, perhaps it is folly to try to hold nurses accountable in so many different ways when they have so little authority. Any discussion of accountability cannot ignore the twin issues of autonomy and authority. This linkage will be discussed in exploring the ramifications of expanding nursing practice and accountability. Despite being used in everyday conversation interchangeably with the word 'responsibility', accountability means something very different and the two words should not be confused. This chapter will therefore address the issue of differentiating between accountability and responsibility.

Accountability and responsibility

The various nursing bodies, tutors and ordinary nurses used to talk a great deal about the responsibilities of being a nurse. It was not the sort of occupation for people lacking a sense of responsibility and duty.

Responsibility means that the nurse is given a charge for which she is answerable. In other words you are given a job or a duty to perform which you are expected to carry out to the best of your ability. There was an implicit assumption that if the nurse did not know how, she would say so rather than carry on and place the patient at hazard. A moment's reflection suggests that nurses have to be responsible in this way and responsibility is therefore a necessary quality for any nurse. The problem comes when it is also seen as a sufficient quality, which was the case from Nightingale's time onwards. Responsibility and a sense of duty chimed nicely with the Victorian order of things when everybody knew their place, which, in the case of women, was doing what they were told, without demur. It is therefore a passive concept in which the nurse waits to be told what to do by either a senior nurse or a doctor.

This historical perspective on the problem of accountability and responsibility has been developed by McCann (1995). She points out that the bruising battle within nursing to establish registration, which culminated in the Nursing Registration Acts of 1919, led to a piece of legislation which divided nursing by setting up supplementary registers (e.g. male nurses, mental nurses, nurses of mental defectives etc.) and left all the decisions of the newly established General Nursing Council (GNC) subject to approval by the Minister of Health and both Houses of Parliament. Nursing was divided and had little absolute control over its affairs with the result that early efforts by the GNC to raise educational standards were thwarted by government interference as it was thought educational standards were being set too high and it would cost too much money. *Plus ça change, plus la même chose* as the French would say! The resulting apprenticeship system of training with its emphasis on obedience and following orders, rather than original thought, led to the growth of responsibility and duty as the main principles guiding nursing practice. As a result of the way nursing was established in the early years of the 20th century, nursing has had no legal status compared to medicine, no professional autonomy, a top heavy system of hierarchy within which the buck could always be passed to somebody else, and a system of apprenticeship training which frowned upon original thinking (McCann, 1995). It is little wonder therefore that duty and responsibility were all and accountability remained an alien concept until very recently.

Accountability was first introduced to nursing as a major theme in the 1992 version of the *UKCC Code of Professional Conduct* and the *Scope of Professional Practice* (UKCC, 1992). There are various definitions of the concept and perhaps the easiest way is think of the word from which accountability is derived, i.e. 'account'. Put simply, accountability means being able to give an account of your actions, to explain and justify why you did what you did. Jones (1996) sees it as encompassing responsibility for one's own actions and also being answerable for them. Rumsey (1997) expands on this simple concept by explaining that accountability involves:

❑ Assessing what is in the best interests of patients in sometimes complex situations

❏ Using nursing knowledge and your own judgement to decide
    upon a course of action
❏ Being able to explain and, if necessary, defend your course of
    action.

Accountability therefore involves responsibility, knowledge and being
able to justify your actions. It also involves the ability to make decisions
and carry them through into practice, i.e. autonomy and authority. It is
therefore a complex concept and one which would have been unthinkable
until recently given what we know of nursing history (McCann, 1995).
The issue of authority has, however, not been emphasized by the UKCC
in their work on accountability and Hancock (1997) points out this
glaring omission from documents such as Scope and the Code of
Conduct. Hancock develops the argument further as she considers that at
present there are areas where nurses cannot be held accountable as they
are not involved in the decision making process. She cites the example of
decisions concerning a patient's resuscitation status; this is still made
usually by the medical staff without nursing input. The UKCC's brave
words about accountability will count for nothing if institutions remain
locked into fragmented and ritualistic approaches to practice, traditional
power structures and controlling hierarchies (Hancock, 1997).

Accountability means that nurses:

❏ Are responsible for their actions at all times
❏ Can justify and explain their actions
❏ Have the authority to act in the way that they think is best for
    the patient.

Accountability, authority and autonomous practice

Hancock's criticism is well directed as authority lies at the heart of any
debate about accountability. Nursing's subservient role within the NHS
has been analysed by Ford and Walsh (1994) who drew upon the writings
of both feminists and critical social theorists to argue that nursing
constitutes an oppressed group with relatively little power and hence
authority. Subsequent work by Parker (1995) continues the theme as she
argues that the relationships and structures which govern the distribution
of power within hospitals only emphasize the disempowerment of
nursing which becomes invisible as a result. It is the privileged status of
medical power and knowledge that is the dominant force within health
care, leaving nursing lacking in power and recognition. This view
challenges the UKCC's assertion that nurses are always accountable as it

is difficult to see how a nurse can be held accountable for something over which she has little or no authority. There is research evidence to support these views as Adamson *et al.* (1995) were able to show high levels of dissatisfaction among their sample of both UK and Australian hospital nurses, based upon perceptions of structural medical dominance and nursing's own lack of power and authority.

Any discussion of accountability must therefore recognize the problem of authority that faces nursing as a whole and the individual nurse in everyday practice. One of the key attributes of accountability is that it is very personal and individualistic. The rise of accountability in nursing came at the end of a period in British political history when the individual was paramount and society took second place. This Thatcherite creed of the 1980s spilled over into the 1990s when both the Scope document and the revised Code of Professional Conduct were being drafted by the UKCC. The linkage between the rise of accountability and the right wing political dogma of Thatcherism is probably not coincidental. When John Major took over from Mrs Thatcher as Prime Minister we were greeted with the named nurse initiative and the notion that every patient should have a nurse named as being responsible for their nursing care. This was a continuation of the same ideology. The named nurse initiative was compromised from the beginning by inadequate staffing levels; nurses' perceived lack of authority to act effectively on behalf of individual patients; lack of ownership of what was another top-down change; and a failure to explore fully what the concept meant, particularly in relation to associate nurses and the concept of primary nursing. These issues are reflected in the findings of Dooley (1999) whose small-scale study was handicapped by a poor response rate, but at least is one of the few attempts actually to research what nurses felt about the named nurse.

Accountability can make the contribution of each individual nurse visible. It is therefore necessary to have a clear view of what the goals are for each individual nurse and nursing team. Nurses cannot be held accountable unless there are unambiguous outcomes and standards against which performance can be measured. Clinical audit is therefore a key component of accountability, especially when linked to critical pathways or as Duff (1995) suggests the dynamic standard setting system (DySSSy). The DySSSy approach emphasizes the importance of nurses setting their own standards for care utilizing the familiar framework of structure, process and outcome. Criteria can then be derived to reflect these standards. The criteria are audited to measure progress towards achieving the agreed standards. Duff argues that as DySSSy allows nurses to set their own standards for nursing care which they can audit, it allows nursing to practice self-regulation and hence accountability. However, the real world of health care does not fall into neat compartments, one of which can be labelled 'nursing'. Health care is a complicated business with many practitioners all influencing patient care. This poses the question of how much care can be isolated for which nurses can be held solely accountable? It also links with the question of authority, for if nurses lack authority, can they be held accountable for failing to achieve certain goals?

There are further complications that Duff (1995) points out. She states that there are two approaches to quality assurance (QA); the traditional

one which seeks to improve quality by removing poor performers, and the practitioner-based approach (e.g. DySSSy) by which nurses pursue their own route to quality improvement by clinicians'own initiatives. If we still work with the traditional model then the emphasis is on institutional control of nursing which, in turn, will lead to suspicion and defensiveness concerning any QA initiatives. Nurses will see QA and talk of personal accountability as tools of management control which can be used to dismiss individuals rather than as positive concepts which can improve patient care and enhance nursing's professional status. Patient complaints are another example of nurses reacting negatively to a potential quality improvement opportunity. Fear of disciplinary action by management makes it a daunting prospect to deal openly and honestly with a complaint. However, as Culley (1998) rightly observes, complaints dealt with constructively can only help drive standards up. This needs an atmosphere of mutual support and understanding among the clinical team and management. Fear of a harsh disciplinary approach and a culture of blame will only cause internal dissent and buck-passing rather than a willingness to admit what went wrong and work to ensuring the same mistake cannot be repeated.

As an example of some of these points, consider the issue of whether hospital nurses can be held accountable for the incidence of pressure sores. An obvious answer is yes. However, it is not that simple as Harrison *et al.* (1998) reported in their account of implementing evidence-based practice. In order to begin a nursing initiative on pressure sores there first has to be agreement upon what constitutes a pressure sore and how they will be measured and graded. A system then has to be introduced for monitoring their incidence. A hospital-wide strategy was necessary and this depended upon the agreement of various other professional groups and ancillary services such as the laundry and portering services. Barriers to change had to be identified and overcome where they could (which was not always possible). Communication had to be established with all the stakeholders in the project in user-friendly language that all could understand. The implementation of that strategy depended upon enough staff being available for release from the wards for training. All staff had to be persuaded of the need to take up the evidence-based guidelines. Wards had to be adequately staffed to allow guidelines to be followed. Where nurses deemed special aids necessary the hospital had to release the resources to make them available. The evidence-based views of the nursing staff concerning dressings for pressure sores that are present have to be paramount. They cannot be overturned by the whim of an individual. The account of Harrison *et al.* paints a picture of major and incremental institutional change over a period of 5 years to achieve implementation of evidence-based guide-lines. A significant reduction in pressure sore incidence has been achieved but only after a massive effort across the whole hospital by all staff.

This example serves to illustrate another point. There is a temptation apparent in the UK during the 1990s to adopt a league table mentality in holding public services accountable for their actions. Teaching in particular has suffered from this problem. Accountability does not mean having a league table based on the incidence of pressure sores by ward or even individual named nurse. This 'name and shame' approach can be very destructive. It is also an invalid exercise as there are many intervening variables that have to be taken into account, such as the condition of the patients and prevalence of pressure sores among the patient population on admission.

This hospital-based example shows many of the problems. Consider now a primary health care example reported by Tinkler *et al.* (1999) in which a team of nurses introduced evidence-based guidelines for the management of leg ulcers in the community. These authors reported that, although there was a strong evidence base to support moving to simple dressings and the use of three or four layer compression bandage systems, their efforts to introduce these changes were hindered by the following factors:

❑ Key components of the effective bandage systems were not available on prescription (orthopaedic wool padding, shaped tubular bandages and cohesive bandages). The health authority made available £55 000 per year purely to meet these extra costs. If the NHS will not make this extra funding available, nurses' attempts to introduce evidence-based care in the management of leg ulcers will be prevented.
❑ Some general practitioners refused to allow 'their nurses' to treat patients who did not belong to the practice with the bandaging regimen in locally organized leg ulcer clinics.
❑ Hospital nurses from wards where patients would be admitted with co-morbidity problems were not released to attend training sessions on the new evidence-based bandaging systems.

Can Tinkler and her colleagues, or other nurses elsewhere engaged on a similar project, be held *fully* accountable for the implementation of evidence-based guidelines if the NHS will not fully fund the work, GPs will not cooperate and hospital wards will not or cannot collaborate in training their own staff? The twin issues of the influence of others and lack of authority illustrated in these two examples indicate that even when there are unambiguous goals, holding nurses *fully* accountable may not be practical due to the effect of intervening variables. This is not, however, an excuse for nurses to say they cannot be held accountable for *anything* as that is tantamount to saying nursing makes no difference to patient outcomes. It is only a short step from there to ask why do we need nurses if they make no difference?

Autonomous practice

If we support the notion of being fully accountable, then there has to be a large degree of autonomy in the way in which nurses practise. There is debate as to whether autonomous means the same as independent practice. The Oxford English Dictionary (1990) defines autonomous as 'having self-government or acting independently'. The nursing profession as a body has a large degree of autonomy already in that it is largely self-governing. In order to explore the second definition it is essential to ask what independence means. According to the Oxford English Dictionary being independent can mean one of three things:

- ❏ Not depending upon the authority or control of others
- ❏ Not depending upon others for earning one's livelihood
- ❏ Being self-governing.

Traditional nursing practice has always depended upon the authority and control of others, i.e. the medical profession and NHS management, so in that sense the individual nurse is not an independent practitioner and therefore not autonomous either. Nurses have always depended upon their employers for a salary, so are not independent in the second sense of the word. The third definition defines independence in terms of autonomy, so from this point of view the two terms do mean the same. This analysis suggests that nursing collectively is a profession that enjoys a high level of autonomy/independence. However, for the individual nurse this is not so as it is the element of control and authority of others that defines independent and hence autonomous practice. Traditionally nurses have perceived themselves as having little control over their own practice and as being subject to the authority of others, hence the view that nursing lacks independence and autonomy.

A moment's reflection will show, however, that it is not possible for any practitioner in the NHS to achieve 100% independence and hence autonomy. Parliament ultimately governs the NHS as a result of funds voted in the Chancellor's Budget, laws passed and reorganizations planned. There is a chain of command from the Department of Health, (and devolved authorities in Scotland, Wales and N. Ireland) and the NHS Executive in England on down to NHS Trusts and Primary Care Groups. National bodies such as the UKCC, GMC, medical Royal Colleges, and the RCN exert a great deal of influence over the individual practitioner whatever their professional grouping. Practitioners have to work in teams and collaborate with other clinicians while patients increasingly have a say in their treatment. In this complex world of modern health care, no clinician can be totally independent. Autonomy is therefore a relative term and nurses might do better to talk of *increasing their level of autonomy*, rather than striving for autonomous practice as the former is realistic and achievable while the latter is not.

Mitchinson (1996) has attempted to separate autonomous from independent practice. She sees the freedom to exercise professional judgement as the cornerstone of autonomous practice while independent practice is characterized by the absence of supervision. Autonomous practice is defined in terms of accountability as Mitchinson sees autonomous practice as:

'. . . defined, negotiated and developed by individual practitioners who are solely responsible and accountable to the patient and to their professional body for their actions and omissions.'

Independent practice is then seen as working with less freedom to define practice than autonomous practice. To practise independently is therefore to reduce the degree of supervision to which the nurse is subject, while autonomous practice largely eliminates supervision. To define anything by the absence of something is not very helpful, yet this is what Mitchinson is doing in her definitions. Mitchinson's paper also uses the terms expanded and extended roles interchangeably which is confusing as they are very different (see p. 51). Her attempts to separate independent and autonomous practice are not helpful, especially as this approach seems to imply they are all or nothing concepts, rather than a question of degree. The Oxford English Dictionary does not differentiate them as it defines each in terms of the other. Perhaps the most useful aspect of this discussion is the attention drawn to the role of clinical judgement and supervision by Mitchinson. If we accept that there is little difference between independent and autonomous practice when seen from the individual nurse's perspective, we can use the degree of freedom to employ clinical judgement as a useful indicator of the degree of autonomy involved. However, the crucial point is the power to act upon that judgement, for if the nurse is not empowered to act, then there is little autonomous practice possible. Supervision implies monitoring and control of practice and in that sense is the mirror image of authority, the more supervision there is the less authority the nurse has. The term can also be used to mean something different as in clinical supervision however, clarity of definition is therefore essential.

The term clinical judgement needs some explanation. The emphasis upon evidence-based health care has given rise to considerable debate concerning the basis for practice in both nursing and medicine. This was explored in the preceding chapter when the legal implications were discussed. Nursing has confounded the issue by talking about intuition as a legitimate basis for expert nursing (Benner, 1984). Walsh (1997) rejects the notion of intuition as the basis for nursing care on the grounds that if called upon to justify your actions (i.e. be accountable), hard evidence will be the yardstick in a court of law

> 'The nurse must be able to justify his or her actions with reference to an objective evidence base if he or she is to earn the authority that will make for truly accountable practice.'

The nurse must therefore have evidence to rely on and be able to show a rational decision making process which led to the chosen course of action. That is not to exclude experience as a source of evidence for the combination of reflection and experience is a valuable learning tool by which we all advance practice. This combination of objective evidence, learning from experience and good decision making skills combine to make clinical judgement which can be used as a basis for practice which enjoys a high degree of autonomy. What many nurses call intuition is actually pattern recognition and a good grasp of the whole which enables the nurse to recognize things are going wrong before he or she can objectively state why.

This discussion brings up a further point about accountability. Not only is it personal and requires clearly measurable goals, but it also involves a two-way contract. Those who are holding nurses accountable must remember their half of the bargain and make the resources and authority available to the nurse to allow him or her to function in an accountable manner.

This issue has been expanded upon by Chalmers (1995) who states that accountability thrives among groups of staff where there is a strong knowledge base, high levels of skill and a commitment to improving standards. Nursing might therefore be considered to fit Chalmer's definition. However, she adds a final and very important point which is that there must also be the maturity to tackle difficult decisions knowing that there will be management and peer support. There must therefore be an atmosphere of support, challenge, encouragement, mutual respect and trust. The relationship between senior NHS management and clinical nurses has not been characterized by mutual respect and trust over the last decade or so. Many nurses feel demotivated, undervalued and unappreciated by management and, at the same time, patronized by the politicians responsible for the NHS.

Nursing itself does not have a good history of 'caring for the carers'. Fletcher (1997) has described the destructive criticism and hostility which has greeted undergraduate and Project 2000 students as well as junior registered nurses who speak out and try to change things for the better. The lack of mutual support among nurses is highlighted in an anecdote told by Nelson (1991). She has described the story of how fishermen in the Carolinas are often asked why they do not bother to put a lid on a fresh caught bucket of crabs. The answer is that if one tries to climb out of the bucket another will catch its leg and pull it back down. Nelson used this as a metaphor for nursing at the start of the 1990s and at the end of the decade her story still has resonance. This is particularly striking when she contrasts the behaviour of crabs with the intelligent, coordinated and mutually supportive behaviour of schools of dolphins! At times nurses are their own worst enemy as they do not support and help each other in the way they should. For example, my own involvement with the Royal College of Nursing Institute BSc Nurse Practitioner course suggests that nurse practitioners who are trying to introduce new and expanded ways of working often face more opposition from fellow nurses than from doctors. If Chalmers is correct about the conditions needed for accountability to flourish, nursing faces a relationship problem within its own ranks and with senior NHS management that could adversely affect the development of true accountability.

Clinical governance

There is a possible way out of this problem and it is provided by the clinical governance agenda introduced by the Labour government after its 1997 General Election victory. Clinical governance links directly into the issues raised above especially the point about management and the managed having a more open and equal relationship. We will therefore briefly explore what clinical governance means before returning to this point.

Clinical governance places a responsibility on each practitioner for their own individual care while emphasizing the importance of quality, consistency and responsiveness (Wilson, 1998). Three key areas are identified by Wilson and accountability is a major theme in each:

❏ Corporate accountability places the Chief Executive in the role of being personally accountable for the performance of the whole NHS Trust. This requires the setting up within the Trust of clear lines of responsibility and accountability.
❏ Internal mechanisms including the emphasis upon individual accountability and self/professional regulation. The increasing emphasis upon staff as life-long learners responsible for continually developing their practice has major implications for education. The NHS has been reluctant to invest substantially in the continuing education of nurses, as many individuals have to pay their own way through courses studied in their own time. Education providers also need to look at the relevance to practice of many of the courses they offer. A good example might be the ENB 997/8 Teaching and Assessing in Practice. It is questionable whether the time and resources consumed by this course make any impact upon clinical outcomes. Educationalists need a broader and more thoughtful approach than just a succession of modules and courses if they are to support the development of clinical practice.
❏ External mechanisms such as the Commission for Health Improvement (CHIMP). This statutory body will police the implementation of clinical governance and therefore will, in one sense, be holding all health service staff accountable for their actions. Additionally, CHIMP is envisaged as having a support and leadership role.

Clinical governance aims to set up a formal framework in which different health professionals can work together to audit and monitor quality of care. Senior management can seek to improve quality and achieve results by hierarchical organizational methods involving incentives (rewards and punishments) and a familiar top-down management style. However, there is another approach outlined by Davies and Mannion (1999) which sees senior management and clinical staff working towards greater understanding and sharing of organizational ends, means and the relationships between them. Mutual trust building measures involving staff and management can lead to greatly enhanced clinical staff performance as practitioners feel that management become less remote and coercive. More recognition by management of practitioners' problems and a willingness to share information and work towards common objectives would reap dividends. This approach contrasts with the confrontational, macho management style that characterized the NHS in the early 1990s at the height of the internal market approach.

Davies and Mannion (1999) conclude their analysis of clinical govern-ance by observing that clinical governance puts quality of care on an equal footing with the financial bottom line in NHS Trust discussions. It represents a major challenge to senior NHS management who, in the aftermath of tragic failures such as that at the Bristol Royal Infirmary, may respond by following a path of ever increasing measurement, stricter monitoring and tighter control. However, these are expensive strategies and Davies and Mannion argue that correcting the current asymmetry in information between management and managed, followed by greater mutual understanding and trust, will lead to major quality gains. Embedded in this idea are the concepts of accountability and self-regulation. Nurses are accountable and must show they can be trusted to regulate their own practice safely. It is encouraging for nursing that accountability and self-regulation are the two key principles that underpin the UKCC Scope document. Nurses are therefore in a strong position to embrace clinical governance providing mutual trust between managers and nurses lies at the heart of future practice. Role expansion should therefore only take place within professionally agreed guidelines and must be underpinned by education and support mechanisms at all times. Under these circumstances nursing can move forward with other professional groups and senior management without the need for coercive restrictive management strategies.

Success in the clinical governance framework therefore depends upon avoiding a culture of blame, instead developing openness, mutual understanding and support as staff work together (Scott, 1998). We have already argued that a more open and equal relationship between senior management and practitioners was essential for accountability. It there-fore follows that clinical governance and accountability go hand in hand.

The key principles embedded in accountability are therefore that it is:

❏ Personal
❏ Involves measurable goals
❏ Requires mutual trust and a more equal relationship between the mangers and the managed.

Accountability and the problem of gravity

Once the principle of accountability is established, it is important to ask accountable to whom? Accountability can be likened to gravity. It is an invisible but powerful force exerted in well-defined directions towards various bodies. The strength of a gravitational force depends (among other things) upon the proximity of the body exerting it. The analogy of accountability as gravity also holds in this respect as the UKCC is seen as remote and distant. The clinical situation, however, in which the doctor asks the nurse to do something or a patient is in distress, is close up and exerts a greater influence upon the nurse's behaviour.

There are three obvious bodies all of whom pull on the nurse's accountability (see Figure 6.1). These are the patient, the employer, the UKCC (and of course the nurse's own conscience). It is possible to extend this list. Watson (1995) adds the medical profession and also introduces accountability into the world of nursing education. The clinical governance agenda reminds nurses they are also accountable to other health professionals besides medicine. With so many different lines of accountability it is likely that there will be times when the nurse finds herself pulled in several different directions at once with mutually contradictory forces at work. An analysis of the lines of accountability faced by the nurse is therefore needed.

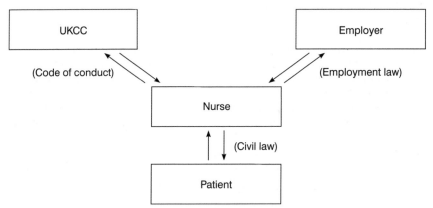

Figure 6.1 Patterns of accountability. The arrows show the two way nature of accountability. The possible involvement of the law is shown in brackets. Nurses are also accountable through the process of critical reflection on practice and ultimately their own conscience

The nurse is held accountable to the patient for the quality of care delivered by the mechanism of civil law. The nurse owes a duty of care to the patient and any breach of that duty which results in harm constitutes negligence for which the patient may seek compensation in the form of damages (see Chapter 5). The patient's family will also hold the nurse accountable for care given and this becomes more significant as the patient becomes less able to speak for himself such as in the case of an elderly patient with dementia or a seriously brain-damaged young adult. The nurse is also accountable to the employer for practice. Employer accountability is regulated through documents such as a job description and contract of employment, together with guidelines and protocols agreed with the employer. The employer exerts sanctions against the nurse through internal disciplinary procedures culminating in dismissal for the most serious offences. The UKCC hold the nurse accountable through the *Code of Professional Conduct* and a series of other documents of which Scope is perhaps the most important. The UKCC also has a range of sanctions at its disposal; the most serious of which is to remove the nurse from the register. The nurse has to go home at the end of the day and sleep with his or her own conscience. This personal accountability has become formalized with the concept of the reflective practitioner, as nurses are encouraged to reflect critically upon their practice in order that they may learn and improve practice.

Other groups of staff such as the medical profession may hold the nurse accountable as Watson (1995) has suggested. Traditionally, doctors have always held nurses *responsible* for carrying out medical instructions concerning their patient, i.e. the doctor's patient. It is open to question whether all doctors have fully grasped the implications of nursing being *accountable* as Watson suggests, rather than responsible in the traditional sense. The knowledge and authority that go alongside genuine accountability may lead to the nurse challenging the doctor's plan of action. If a genuine exchange of views and discussion takes place, leading to agreement about the way forward, that is indeed accountable practice. However, if doctors merely brush aside nursing suggestions or challenges, claiming medical prerogative and authority, then that can hardly be seen as the nurse accountable to the doctor. We have also explored the concept that accountability is a 'two way street' (p. 95) which leads to the conclusion that there is a way in which the doctor would also be accountable to the nurse if there were true accountability. This opens up a fascinating line of thought; how can we hold doctors accountable for the quality of their medical care? It may be that other staff such as paramedics, therapists or social workers view the nurse in a more accountable light than doctors.

The problem for nurses is that these lines of accountability may cross and at times go in opposite directions, leaving the nurse with a serious dilemma as to which course of action to take. Most nurses will have faced the situation where staffing is short and there is a lot of pressure from some very sick patients. Things become so bad that you feel patient safety is compromised and you are all too aware of the UKCC strictures about safe practice. However, pulling in the opposite direction is your employer who merely tells you things are tough, the Trust cannot afford or find any more staff so you will just have to get on with it and do the best you can. Medical staff may be eroding your time further by expecting you to take bloods and give IV medication. This familiar situation leaves the nurse with two sets of forces pulling in opposite directions along opposite lines of accountability. At the heart of this tug of war is the nurse trying to decide what to do and be accountable to him- or herself in the process. Do you do the best you can and hope nothing goes wrong which will put you in front of the UKCC or in court? Do you refuse to do medical work and go to the press in the desperate hope that publicity might force your employers to do something, risking disciplinary action and dismissal in the process?

Clause 1 of the *UKCC Code of Conduct* (UKCC, 1992) states that in the exercise of professional accountability each nurse shall:

'Act always in such a way as to promote and safeguard the wellbeing and interests of patients/clients'.

This is a strong statement. However, when the nurse encounters the sort of situation described in the preceding paragraph and looks to the Code to find out how he or she is supposed to achieve the aim of clause 1, she finds clause 10 advising her

> '. . . to make known to appropriate persons or authorities any circumstances which could place patients/clients in jeopardy or which militate against safe standards of practice'.

The UKCC does not appear to expect the nurse to take any direct action but merely to inform a senior person that things are not safe.

This could be seen as unhelpful and ineffective advice or seen pragmatically as the UKCC acknowledging that actually there is very little the nurse can do about the real world of clinical practice. If the former is the case then the UKCC is a toothless tiger and its *Code of Conduct* as much use as the famous piece of paper that Chamberlain brought back from Munich in 1938 which was supposed to represent 'peace in our time'. If the UKCC is merely being pragmatic and acknowledging the relative powerlessness of nurses, it is difficult to see how they can justify basing the entire *Code of Conduct* on the assumption that the nurse is personally accountable for each of the 14 clauses it contains? Perhaps it is time for the *Code of Professional Conduct* to receive an overhaul that addresses this fundamental question of accountability without authority. Clinical governance alone will demand that there have to be changes made to the Code as it places much greater emphasis upon individual practitioners. Simply telling a senior person that care is not safe may not be seen as an adequate response if Trusts are required to set stringent quality improvement targets under the requirements of clinical governance.

The issue that lies at the heart of this situation is one of authority and power. Crises relating to staffing and the quality of care usually arise because of senior management's preoccupation with the financial position of the Trust rather than the quality of care given and an unwillingness to try to find new ways of working which make more effective use of what staff is available. If clinical governance is more than just another slogan, but actually leads to real changes in the way the NHS works, then situations such as these should become less frequent. The key point made by Hancock (1997) that the UKCC documents lack recognition of the disempowered position of nurses also comes to the fore as in this situation nurses are powerless to change anything.

There are many other situations where the nurse finds the forces of accountability pulling in different directions. One of the most complex concerns the problem presented by the patient whose expectations of care are at odds with what the nurse knows is professionally best practice and may also be at odds with what the family wants. The notion of patient as partner in care has received a lot of attention recently (see Chapter 1), however, the nurse may find that the overweight, unfit, hypertensive individual who smokes 30 a day and who has a most unhealthy diet refuses to change any of these habits. Health education advice falls on deaf ears and may lead to conflict with the patient who robustly informs you that his father smoked 30 a day and did not pay any attention to all these health scares and it never did him any harm. Patients with other chronic diseases such as diabetes or renal failure also fall into this category while community psychiatric nurses also face the same problem but in a different context. Non-cooperation by the patient with lifestyle modifications and medication regimens will have serious detrimental consequences. The nurse is the only potential continual health service contact and as such is in the best position to monitor progress and hopefully change behaviours, hence the importance of maintaining contact.

The problem is that in pursuing what you see as the best interests of the patient by attempting to negotiate lifestyle change you may find yourself in conflict with him and his family leading to a complete breakdown in care. Is the patient always right even when they are wrong? A more extreme scenario might be the patient who is determined to commit suicide either as a result of depression or a terminal illness such as motor neurone disease or cancer. The patients' rights and our commitment to put the patients' wishes first now lead us into a position where, if we materially assisted his death in any way, we would be in breach of the criminal law. Even if we did not actively assist in suicide, how might the UKCC respond to a nurse openly stating that the patient should be allowed to end his life and arguing that cause as patient advocate? The nurse could be argued in that situation to be in breach of a duty of care owed to the patient and therefore open to civil proceedings for negligence if harm subsequently occurred. Issues such as these question the notion of the nurse as patient advocate Expanding nursing roles, as I shall argue later, also adds a new series of challenges to the validity of this concept.

Advocacy

Advocacy is simply defined by McMillan and Townsend (1994) as having a concern for your client's rights and being active in protecting those rights, even though this may bring you into conflict with other members of the health care team. This requires assertiveness on the part of the nurse and a willingness to be unpopular. The nurse as advocate role is easy to recognize in clinical situations such as dealing with pain as the nurse is ideally placed to monitor and control the patient's pain, obtaining changes to prescriptions from medical staff as necessary. Even the novice nurse can contribute towards nursing advocacy as he or she can make the necessary observations about pain levels even if it requires a more expert nurse to understand their significance and act accordingly (Fordham and Dunn, 1994).

There is however more to advocacy than the notion of speaking out for the patient for, as Tschudin (1992) reminds us, advocacy should be based upon the patient's needs not the nurse's wants or desires. If nurses can separate off their own wants and desires this still leaves the problem of the patient's *needs*. What the patient expresses as a need may be a want or a desire which is not essential to care or which may actually be very harmful to care. It may also be based upon prejudice or ignorance such as the racist who demands to be moved from his bed because it is next to a black patient. Would the nurse advocate for that patient and in the process support racism? Consider the patient with peripheral vascular disease who insists on smoking, will the nurse advocate for him to be allowed to smoke in the day room to the discomfort and harm of everybody else in addition to himself? The nurse is faced with the difficult task of disentangling what the patient needs from what the patient wants or desires and in the process may find herself influencing the patient in such a way that she is no longer acting as advocate.

It follows from this analysis that to be an advocate the nurse has fully to understand the patient and there has to be dialogue between the two. Kendrick (1998) addressed these issues in a paper he delivered at the national RCN A&E conference in 1998. He pointed out that many nurses only have very short patient consultations (e.g. the A&E nurse or Practice Nurse) and as a result there is insufficient time to understand the patient's motives, desires, wants and needs. It is difficult to have a dialogue with many patients such as those who are aggressive, under the influence of alcohol, unconscious, dementing or who do not speak English as a natural first language. Kendrick also asked the nurse how she would feel advocating for a terrorist, a neo-Nazi racist thug or a man who had just severely beaten his wife? Perhaps advocacy under those circumstances is best left to the professional advocates, i.e. the legal profession. Advocacy, according to Kendrick, cannot therefore be seen as a general principle applicable to all patients. Rather there are soft easy areas such as the patient in pain referred to above, but there are many other areas where it is not realistic.

A further problem with Tschudin's argument is that the nurse may actually want or desire to practise evidence-based care which is acknowledged as best practice. The logic of the nurse as advocate role is that he or she should be prepared to set aside evidence-based best practice in order to comply with the patient's wishes, which may well be *perceived* as needs by the patient. Negotiation with the patient may well lead to evidence-based care winning the day and the patient cooperating with treatment. However, it may not, which is when the nurse as advocate role becomes untenable as it leaves the nurse's lines of professional accountability to her employer, the UKCC, medical staff pulling in the opposite direction. It also leaves you with the dilemma of reflecting upon your own practice which you know is not helping the patient and may be doing harm, even if it is making the patient happy in the short term.

The discussion about advocacy also has to be placed in the context of existing power structures within the NHS. As we have already seen nurses are relatively disempowered and while they might speak out for patients, nobody may be listening. The power to make decisions about the important aspects of care traditionally lies elsewhere. Doctors see individual clinical matters as their domain and managers decide whether the doctors will have a ward or unit in which to make clinical decisions at all. In such an environment, nurses can quickly become frustrated and disillusioned if they try to act as patient advocates and may quickly become labelled as trouble makers.

One of the consequences of the nurse moving into more autonomous and expanded roles is that she will have more authority in clinical decision making. This may be thought to open the door to a more positive advocacy role as the power of others is diminished. There is a problem lurking here, however, against whom does the nurse advocate? The nurse practitioner may see the patient with an undifferentiated and undiagnosed problem, arrive at a diagnosis as a result of history taking and examination skills and then seek to implement a course of therapeutic action. Consider now the situation where the patient disagrees or is unwilling to cooperate with treatment. This leaves the nurse to advocate on behalf of the patient against the person directing care, i.e. herself! As it is not possible to advocate against yourself, this calls into question the whole concept of advocacy as part of expanded nursing roles such as the nurse practitioner.

The previous example shows the nurse practitioner using extra knowledge and skills to make decisions about treatment based upon best evidence and practice. Negotiation and explanation will often bring about patient cooperation, although this could already be argued to have crossed the boundary of advocacy as the nurse is working actively to persuade the patient to follow her recommended course of action. The nurse is held accountable by the employer for her actions and will also have to satisfy the medical profession that she is working in her expanded role within guidelines for best practice. The UKCC are also holding her accountable for the delivery of care that is in the patient's best interests. The combined gravitational pull of accountability to these bodies makes it imperative that the nurse delivers care that she knows represents evidence-based best practice. If the patient is unwilling to cooperate, she has no choice other than to try to explain, persuade and negotiate with the patient to achieve these outcomes. Advocacy under these circumstances is simply not possible.

This issue was anticipated by Walsh (1985) who observed that nurses will always be concerned about their jobs and the needs of their employer, so much so that their role as advocate is fatally compromised. Porter (1988) also observed that as nurses work within the health care system, they have a vested interest in maintaining that system and the place of the patient within it. Advocacy can only ever be a form of 'benign paternalism' according to Porter as anything else would undermine the power and authority that all health care staff hold over patients.

This discussion of advocacy and the nurse's accountability to the patient suggests that while you must always abide by the UKCC *Code of Conduct* and put the patient's interests first, you may find real dilemmas caused by the gravity-like pull exerted by accountability to other bodies. The notion of nurse as patient advocate has serious problems and there are many situations where it is not practical. Accountability to employers and doctors undermines advocacy, while the development of increasingly autonomous roles may leave the nurse having to advocate against herself as the clinician accountable for the patient's care.

Summary

This chapter has reviewed the concept of accountability, noting that it is a relative newcomer to the nursing lexicon. The ability to give an account of your actions and justify practice lies at the heart of accountability. This however requires sound knowledge and evidence-based practice together with the authority to act in accordance with best evidence. The accountable nurse therefore has to enjoy a significant degree of autonomy, a point that the UKCC does not appear to have taken fully on board in its statements about accountability. A useful analogy for understanding accountability is provided by the force of gravity as each body in the universe exerts a pull upon the nurse but in different directions and proportional to its distance. The nurse may therefore find herself pulled in different directions at once, caught between the strength of the immediate clinical situation and the distant pull of bodies such as the UKCC. This chapter concludes by questioning the conventional wisdom of the nurse as patient advocate as there are many patients for whom the nurse cannot advocate. Increasing autonomy and the associated accountability that go with more expanded roles also lead to the conclusion that nurses working in such advanced roles cannot act as patient advocates as they may have to advocate against themselves.

References

Adamson, B. J., Kenny, D. T. and Wilson-Barnett, J. (1995). The impact of perceived medical dominance on workplace satisfaction of Australian and British nurses. *Journal of Advanced Nursing*, **21**, 172–183.

Benner, P. (1984). *From Novice To Expert*. Menlo Park CA: Addison Wesley.

Chalmers, H. (1995). Accountability in nursing models and the nursing process. In: Watson, R. (ed.) *Accountability in Nursing Practice*. London: Chapman Hall.

Culley, F. (1998). Tissue viability: the facts and the law. *Nursing Times*, **94**, 24, 63–64.

Davies, H.T. and Mannion, R. (1999). *Clinical Governance: Striking a Balance Between Checking and Trusting. Discussion paper 165*. York: University of York, Centre for Health Economics.

Dooley, F. (1999). The named nurse in practice. *Nursing Standard*, **13**, 34, 33–38.

Duff, L. (1995). Standards of care, quality assurance and accountability. In: Watson, R. (ed.) *Accountability in Nursing Practice*. London: Chapman Hall.

Fletcher, J. (1997). Do nurses really care? Some unwelcome findings from recent research and inquiry. *Journal of Nursing Management*, **5**, 43–50.

Ford, P. and Walsh, M. (1994). *Nursing through the Looking Glass; New Rituals for Old*. Oxford: Butterworth-Heinemann.

Fordham, M. and Dunn, V. (1994). *Alongside the Person in Pain*. London: Bailliere Tindall.

Jones, M. (1996). *Accountability in Practice*. Salisbury: Mark Allen Publishing.

Hancock, H. (1997). Professional responsibility: implications for nursing practice within the realms of cardiothoracics. *Journal of Advanced Nursing*, **25**, 1054–1060.

Harrison, J., Logan, J., Joseph, L. and Graham, I. (1998). Quality improvement, research and evidence based practice: 5 years experience with pressure sores. *Evidence Based Nursing*, **1**, 4, 108–110.

Kendrick, K. (1998). *Advocacy and the A&E Nurse*. RCN A&E Forum Conference, November 1998, Daresbury Hall Centre.

McCann, S. (1995). The development of nursing as an accountable profession. In: Watson, R. (ed.) *Accountability in Nursing Practice*. London: Chapman Hall.

McMillan, M. and Townsend, J. (1994). *Reflections on Contemporary Nursing Practice*. Oxford: Butterworth-Heinemann.

Mitchinson, S. (1996). Are nurses independent and autonomous practitioners? *Nursing Standard*, **10**, 34, 34–38.

Nelson, J. (1991). A crab or a dolphin: a new paradigm for nursing practice. *Nursing Outlook*, **39**, 3, 136–137.

Parker, J. (1995). Searching for the body in nursing. In: Gray, G. and Pratt, R. (eds) *Scholarship in the Discipline of Nursing*. Sydney: Churchill Livingstone.

Porter, S. (1988). Siding with the system. *Nursing Times*, **84**, 14, 30–31.

Rumsey, M. (1997). Nurse accountability. *Practice Nurse*, 21 February 1997, 136–139.

Scott, A. (1998). Clinical governance relies upon a change in culture. *British Journal of Nursing*, **7**, 16, 940.

Tinkler, A., Hotchkiss, J. and Edwards, E. (1999). Implementing evidence based leg ulcer management. *Evidence Based Nursing*, **2**, 1, 6–8.

Tschudin, V. (1992). *Ethics in Nursing* (2nd edn). Oxford: Butterworth-Heinemann.

UKCC (1992). *Code of Professional Conduct*. London: UKCC.

UKCC (1992) *The Scope of Professional Practice*. London: UKCC.

Walsh, P. (1985). Speaking up for the patient. *Nursing Times*, **81**, 18, 24–27.

Walsh, M. (1997). Accountability and intuition: justifying nursing practice. *Nursing Standard*, **11**, 23, 39–41.

Watson, R. (1995). *Accountability in Nursing Practice*. London: Chapman Hall.

Wilson, J. (1998). Clinical governance. *British Journal of Nursing*, **7**, 16, 985–986.

Yeats, W. B. (1921). The Double Vision of Michael Robartes. In: A. N. Jeffares (ed.) *WB Yeats, Selected Poetry*. London: Pan Books.

CHAPTER 7

Expanding the boundaries of nursing practice

No man has a right to fix the boundary of a march of a nation; no man has a right to say to his country – thus far shalt thou go and no further.

Charles Parnell, Cork, 21st January 1885.

Introduction

The message 'thus far and no further' is familiar to many nurses. It seems to be frequently sent out whenever they have tried to develop and expand their practice. It is therefore fitting to open this chapter with the source of that quotation, Charles Parnell. He was one of the great leaders of the Irish nation's struggle for freedom and in his speech at Cork he is clearly making the point that outsiders cannot stop the natural development of a nation. Once a group of people starts acting together in their common interest, they acquire a momentum of their own. As Giroux (1985) observed history is never foreclosed. It is only the product of human behaviour, which is, in turn, open to challenge and change. Human (and therefore nursing) history is consequently open ended, continuous and has no end point other than the extinction of the human species. Nobody has the right to hold back the development of nursing, providing that development is within the law of the land and in the patients' best interests. Statements such as the *UKCC Code of Professional Conduct* and other agreements on human rights by international bodies such as the ICN and UN provide the ethical framework within which nursing can develop. So long as nursing remains within these legal and ethical boundaries, Parnell's ringing declaration is equally valid today. Nobody has the right to say thus far and no further if it can be shown that nursing is moving towards better patient care that is both cost and clinically effective.

Boundaries in an expanding universe

Boundaries are all around us. They are lines of demarcation that help us make sense of the world by separating entities such as territory, occupations or objects from one another. In that sense they are useful. Interprofessional boundaries help patients distinguish between the different health professionals they encounter. This in turn allows the patient to seek the right care and attention from the right person. It also allows health professionals to make sense of the complicated world of health care by being able to allocate different people to different categories of staff and therefore know what their role is in providing care for the patient.

However, people have a habit of using boundaries in a less constructive way. If a person sits within a boundary looking outwards, they may chose to define the area enclosed by the boundary in possessive terms. This is mine, something I am going to hold on to and not share with outsiders. Boundaries then become positions to be defended, lines in the sand that will not be crossed. Barbed wire entanglements are erected, trenches are dug and minefields are laid, metaphorically or literally speaking. Change and various external pressures lead to insecurity and a perception of threat. A siege mentality develops accompanied by hostility to outsiders. In the international world of geopolitics the stage is set for conflict and war. In the world of health care the stage is set for what the Americans call 'a turf war' as different professional groups fight over the control of territory within the health care field.

Boundaries can therefore be seen as very negative and harmful to patient care as they lead to professional groups spending vital time and energy in conflict with each other rather than fighting their common enemy, ill health and disease. They also ossify health care as it is partitioned up in rigid compartments which have far more to do with professional vested self-interest than the welfare of the patient. At times health care resembles the trench warfare of the Western Front in World War I. Large bodies of personnel may become gridlocked in unproductive conflict and mutual suspicion, dug into the entrenched positions that they have occupied for so long that nobody remembers how they got there, why they are there or, most importantly, where they are supposed to be going. Between the trenches is no man's land where any brave soul foolish enough to venture is immediately picked off by the heavy artillery of the other side, while snipers lie in wait for anybody who sticks their head above the parapet.

'That is gross over-exaggeration, relationships with medicine are not that bad', I can hear you say, but who said I was only writing of medicine? Sadly there are times when relationships within nursing degenerate to this level as health visitors and midwives hold themselves separate from nurses, while even the recent reforms of basic nursing education, embodied in project 2000, perpetuated the split of nursing into four different areas. In setting standards for post-registration nursing the UKCC went further as they split primary health care nursing alone into eight different specialities. Nursing has to consider its relationships with other professional groups such as medicine against this background of disunity and internal wrangling.

If we set aside these internal divisions for the time being and admit that the picture painted above is something of a caricature, consideration of the wider field of health care shows that there are strong vested interests determined to defend 'their territory' from perceived incursions by others. Nurses are frequently seen as the interlopers. Should they seek to move on from traditional nursing territory, crossing the boundary into no man's land beyond the last strand of barbed wire marked 'Made in Scutari', they may well attract the heavy artillery of the medical profession. They may also find that radiographers are lobbing mortar bombs in their direction for suggesting that nurses may be able to order X-rays and interpret them. This is despite the fact that a rigorous study by Meek *et al.* (1998) found that A&E nurse practitioners were as competent as experienced senior house officers (SHOs) in interpreting X-rays and were better than inexperienced SHOs. Even sticking a head above the parapet with a simple suggestion to include antibiotics in a group protocol to improve practice in A&E can attract a lethal volley of fire from the hospital pharmacy (Senior, 1999). Community nurses are also very familiar with the potential conflict that can arise with social services in determining the care requirements of patients in their own homes.

Boundaries can be destructive zones of conflict, but that need not be. The problems arise if staff think of their territory as being constant and static. This issue has been introduced in Chapter 4, but such is its importance that we will return to it here. The steady state view of the universe is as old as man's ideas about the nature of things. The Ancient Greeks saw the universe as constant and perfect, a philosophy adopted by Christianity and only challenged when Galileo pointed the first telescopes at the sky in the early 17th century. He saw change and imperfection everywhere and got into serious trouble with the Catholic church for saying so. It is much more comfortable to think of our world as being stable and working well. It was in the 17th century and still is now. As health professionals we therefore like to hang on to what we have. We do not want change and we do not want to be told that, as things are not going well, we will have to do things differently to make them better. So we prefer to think of practice as a stable, steady state. To help explore this problem further, in Chapter 4 we visualized the field of health care as a fixed area, bounded by a drystone wall much as the field that is outside my study window now. One group of animals in that field (nurses) can only expand their area of grazing at the expense of another (doctors). If the area of health care is a constant size, then the only way one group of professionals can expand their practice is at the expense of others, leading to conflict as staff retreat behind their professional boundaries determined to hold on to what they have. This is the conventional way of conceptualizing health care.

In Chapter 4 we borrowed a metaphor from cosmology to see things in a different way. Cosmology teaches that the universe has been in a state of expansion ever since the big bang that brought it into being. Galaxies are therefore moving away from each other, space is expanding as time unravels. Now consider the universe of health care, it too is an expanding universe. With the passage of time medical technology makes greater and greater leaps forward and so new treatments become possible keeping people alive longer. The ageing population leads to ever increasing demands upon health care resources while our complex society spawns new health problems from AIDS to stress-induced illness. Poverty and social disadvantage show no signs of going away and nobody really knows what the effects of climate change will be on global health. These are just a few of the driving forces leading to an expansion in the universe of health care. The closed constant field surrounded by a dry stone wall has gone, replaced by a complex and expanding world of ever increasing health demands and patient expectations. Seen in this way, there is clearly room for individual groups to expand their practice without threatening the territorial integrity of others as the whole field is getting bigger all the time. Boundaries become flexible and moveable but no one group should have to defend their territory against another as the whole field is expanding.

Without role and practice expansion, the health care system will be unable to keep up with the increasing demand for health care. To stay with the cosmological analogy, black holes will begin to appear in the fabric of health care. Patients with unmet needs will fall into these holes and disappear from view. This is especially pertinent when the reduction in the numbers of GPs is considered together with the reduction in the number of junior doctors' hours available for hospital care as a result of the 'New Deal' for junior doctors. Groups of staff such as nurses have to expand their boundaries of practice if we are to even maintain the present far from perfect coverage of the field. Boundary expansion needs also to be accompanied by realignment elsewhere. If medical staff recognize that nurses may take over areas of care that were once the doctors' domain, nursing may have to face the same dilemma and, in the absence of a major increase in the number of registered nurses, we too may have to hand over aspects of care to health care assistants or patients themselves. Such is the rate of expansion of this health care universe that completely new care modalities and associated groups of staff may have to be created to maintain a continuous health care fabric. Perhaps the recent growth in the popularity of complementary therapies and the dramatic development of paramedics may represent such developments?

When boundaries are seen as dynamic areas of interaction, rather than static zones of conflict, a much more positive picture emerges. Inevitably there will be friction as two different substances or cultures rub against each other, but the interaction can be very productive although somewhat unpredictable. Cross-fertilization, whether it be of pollen in the herbaceous border or of ideas in the world of human behaviour, can produce some startling hybrids which are much greater than the mere sum of their parts. This leads to the suggestion that there might be real improvements in patient care if a significant number of nurses embraced some traditional medical skills or doctors combined better approaches to communication with a wider holistic perspective. Nursing has much to teach medicine and vice versa.

Health care is not only an expanding universe but it is also a dynamic system. In the natural sciences the phrase 'a dynamic system' means simply that what happens upstream influences what happens later downstream. There is therefore some kind of feedback mechanism. In systems such as these, sensitive feedback loops mean that small-scale fluctuations can produce very surprising results as a minor disturbance in one place can lead to major and unforeseen complications elsewhere. Such mechanisms are at work in health care, which, by analogy, is a dynamic system. What happens for example in nursing education today effects nursing practice tomorrow. There is interaction between different components of the health care system as developments in medicine often have major implications for nursing and vice versa. Clearly the Conservative government of the 1980s did not consider that reducing the numbers of nurses in training would have a major impact upon the practice of medicine. Five to 10 years later there is a shortage of nurses and the problem of staffing ITU beds with adequate numbers of sufficiently skilled nurses has had a significant and frustrating effect upon the practice of medicine.

There is a striking similarity to this condition in the natural sciences. It is known as chaos theory and put simply it states that if there is sensitive dependence upon initial conditions, then a dynamic system can behave in an apparently unpredictable way, i.e. it appears chaotic. However, within the apparent chaos there are still simple rules governing behaviour, it is not random chance at work. This is because initial minor errors or disturbances can be amplified rapidly by feedback mechanisms operating within the basic rules governing the system (Cohen and Stewart,1994). If we accept the analogy that health care is a dynamic system, then we can argue that it is also chaotic and apparently unpredictable. Nursing therefore needs to be able to adapt to rapid and major changes in health care, some of which may have been triggered off by nurses themselves.

One interesting property of chaotic systems is that boundary regions are particularly prone to sensitive dependence upon initial conditions and therefore it is impossible to draw precise lines that separate one condition from another. Although at a coarse level it is possible to discriminate between two obviously different conditions (e.g. nursing and medicine), in fine detail the boundary vanishes into ever more complicated and unpredictable twists and turns known in chaos theory as fractals. It is a peculiar property of the real world that often when you look at boundaries, no matter what scale you use, their shape is the same. In other words you can view a boundary reduced on a scale of kilometres to the centimetre as on a map and keep taking small sections of the boundary and enlarging them but the shapes keep reproducing them-selves in ever more complex patterns. Sharp boundaries therefore do not exist in nature; there is merely a complicated fractal fuzz. Cohen and Stewart (1994) remind us that it may not be possible to draw a precise boundary that distinguishes between two obviously different extremes such as male and female or dead and alive. We can recognize that Arnold Schwarzenegger or Madonna lie a long way either side of the boundary between male and female, but drawing the line itself is extremely difficult. Human sexuality is far too complicated for a simple division.

So it is with nursing and medicine. We recognize obvious examples of each when we see them (almost stereotypes), but drawing a sharp, clear and unambiguous boundary between nursing and medicine is not possible (Figure 7.1). It is only natural that there will be nurses working in such a way that their practice straddles the boundary with medicine or other professional groups, that is the natural order of things. To try to impose crystal clear lines of demarcation is an artificial exercise that is doomed to failure. However much bureaucrats and institutions may want to divide up health care into neat boxes and place all staff into one box or another, they are unlikely to succeed because reality will intervene. Nurses are embedded in the 'chaotic' system of health care that is carried out by human beings and which does not have simple two-dimensional boundaries.

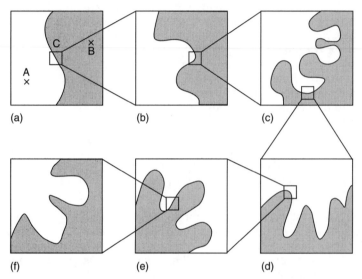

Figure 7.1 This diagram represents the boundary between nursing and medicine and while (a) shows that persons at A and B are clearly a nurse and a doctor, trying to define practice at the boundary in area C in such simple terms is not possible. The fractal nature of boundaries means that no matter how much you enlarge the boundary it always dissolves into more complex details as you move from 1a to 1f. There is no hard and fast boundary, only a zone of complex fractal fuzz where practice could be either nursing or medicine

Drawing analogies with the natural sciences suggests that nurses practising at the boundaries of nursing and medicine are therefore in a grey area where there is no clear line of demarcation and cross-fertilization of ideas and practices can occur. While it is possible to recognize a heart surgeon as obviously a doctor and a nurse working with the terminally ill as obviously a nurse, those who try to impose a single one-dimensional line, unambiguously dividing nursing from medicine, will get it wrong. This is a grey area where unpredictable and major changes can occur very quickly and minor alterations in normal practice can have unforeseen consequences. It is not surprising that cumbersome statutory bodies such as the UKCC find the expanding boundaries of nursing practice very hard to keep up with.

Traditional science has for many centuries been based upon reductionist principles. In order to understand a complex entity, the investigator breaks it down into small pieces and works with these simpler building blocks, hence the term 'reductionism'. This approach has achieved a great deal of success up to a point. The so-called medical model is a good example of this approach as the body is broken down into systems and their component parts leading to medical specialization. It has however become apparent in the closing decades of this century that this approach has reached the limits of its usefulness as a great many problems remain unsolved and apparently insoluble. This is the case in both the natural and social sciences, in which medicine and health are firmly embedded.

Discoveries in the field of chaos have led to a new way of looking at the world which rejects reductionism in favour of recognizing the complexity that surrounds us and trying to work with that complexity. Put simply, the whole is more than the sum of the parts and to understand the world around us we have to look at the interactions between its components rather than break it down into ever smaller subsystems which are then studied in isolation from each other. The overall organization of a system gives it an emergent property, something that does not exist in the bits of the system but only becomes apparent when it is all put together. Movement is an emergent property of the motor car just as life is an emergent property of the bits that make up the human body. The notion that separate systems contribute to higher level characteristics is inherent in Complexity theory and applies to both the biological and social sciences, including nursing (Ray, 1998). As Coveney and Highfield (1995) have said:

> Instead of attempting to take a deterministic, mechanical view of the world, we need a higher level perspective if we are to make sense of it. . . . A human being is an emergent property of huge numbers of cells, a company is more than the sum of its pens, papers, real estate and personnel'
>
> Coveney and Highfield, p. 330

In terms of looking at how we organize health care, we have to move away from wanting to put staff into neat little boxes where they are bound by strict rules and constrained by artificial boundaries. The NHS needs a higher level perspective, especially one that recognizes that it is more than the sum of its equipment, patient records, nursing notes, hospitals, health centres, doctors, nurses, midwives etc., to paraphrase Coveney and Highfield. What makes patient care is the interaction between patients, their surroundings and all the various staff and equipment that make up the NHS. The whole is greater than the sum of its parts and we need to recognize this, adopting a more fluid approach to practice development that is in the patients' best interests, rather than trying to break the NHS down into its constituent building blocks and imposing barriers between them. This reductionist approach leads to a 'This far and no further' mentality rather than a creative interaction between staff patients and their surroundings.

We have discussed practice on the boundaries of nursing in abstract terms. When we look at what is actually happening in the real world we find ample evidence of the sort of fuzzy grey areas that bureaucrats and managers hate. This has been brought to a head by the nurse practitioner movement and we will now explore this development as it can be understood in terms of being an emergent property of health care complexity. Please bear in mind the last few pages as you read on!

Nurse practitioners; complexity and chaos at the boundaries of medicine and nursing

Nurse practitioners (NP) lie at the junction of medicine and nursing. They are at the boundaries of nursing and located within the dynamic system of health care. Chaos theory and the emerging discipline of complexity therefore offer us a framework within which to locate their development. Such a framework can make sense of what is happening and also dispel unnecessary alarms about 'taking over medicine' or 'subordinating nursing to medicine'. Both these mutually exclusive notions have been advanced by opponents of the NP concept, which suggests an illogical and flawed approach to the debate. They cannot both be right!

This discussion is immediately complicated by the fact that there is no official definition of the NP role in the UK as the UKCC has consistently refused to recognize the concept. This has led to a wide range of nurses wearing 'Nurse Practitioner' badges as health providers have adopted the term to describe a very wide range of roles. The concept originated in the USA in the 1970s as a means of making health care accessible to rural populations. Ford and Walsh (1994) charted the rapid and highly successful development of the NP movement in the USA and its early growth in the UK thanks to pioneers such as Barbara Stilwell.

Despite the extensive North American evidence and a series of highly successful pilot studies in the UK, the UKCC has set its face against the NP. Castledine (1995) dismissed NPs as 'an obstacle' to the UKCC Specialist and Advanced nursing proposals contained in the UKCC (1994) *Post-registration Education for Practice* document (PREP) which have since been abandoned. He saw NPs as nurses satisfying their own curiosity and desire to pursue a more medical and technical approach to care. This negative and incorrect assertion is not helpful to the development of any discipline, particularly as there is substantial evidence to the contrary which suggests that NPs work with a holistic health oriented model (Edwards *et al.*, 1999) and are more likely to value the psychosocial aspects of nursing than nurses (Walsh, 1999). Critics of the NP movement also go on to argue that they are merely propagating nursing's subservience to medicine by taking on medical tasks (MacAlister and Chiam, 1995). If nurses passively accept delegated jobs that doctors no longer wish to do, this is a valid criticism. However, correctly defining the NP role ensures that this is not the case and places nurses at the forefront of developing NP practice collaboratively with doctors and patients. The UKCC's failure to embrace the NP concept is therefore only exacerbating the problem.

A simple approach to the problem of definition might be to state that a NP is a nurse who is working with higher levels of autonomy than found in traditional nursing and whose practice is underpinned by appropriate advanced education. A more detailed definition has been provided by the Royal College of Nursing and this underpins the RCN Institute BSc Hons Nurse Practitioner course which is available at a range of higher education institutions across the UK. This may be summarized by saying the NP:

❑ Sees patients with undifferentiated/undiagnosed problems
❑ Makes a health assessment utilizing extra skills not normally taught in nursing education to date
❑ Makes professionally autonomous decisions for which he or she has sole responsibility
❑ Develops a plan of nursing care to promote health
❑ Provides counselling and health education
❑ Screens patients for early signs of illness/risk factors
❑ Has the authority to admit, discharge or refer patients to other health professionals.

The RCN statement adds that the nature of the role is such that it must be supported by education to at least honours degree level (RCN, 1996).

This definition straddles nursing and medicine but is much closer to nursing than it is medicine. There are several key points that distinguish it from conventional nursing however. The NP is the first point of contact for the patient who will often present with a health problem that has not been assessed and diagnosed by a doctor. In primary health care and A&E settings this is obvious. Nurse practitioners are also developing roles in outpatients and surgical specialities where the patient is under a consultant and has a medical diagnosis such as arthritis of the hip or benign hyperplasia of the prostate. The NP role is still valid as when the patient presents, he may bring with him a range of health problems other than the principal clinical diagnosis. The ability of nurses to consider the whole patient rather than focus on a narrow piece of pathology means the NP is well equipped to care for the patient in these circumstances. The NP can therefore manage ongoing care for chronic conditions via the outpatients department (OPD). In addition to having a wider perspective, he or she will provide much greater continuity of care than traditional medical practice as patients often see a different doctor every time they attend OPD. The width of vision associated with the NP role also makes it ideal for running a preoperative assessment clinic. Such a clinic can avoid admitting patients who are not fit for surgery or those whose condition has changed such that they no longer need surgery. The NP can also start planning for discharge before admission. This latter point is particularly important in dealing with elderly patients who may need substantial social and nursing support for a safe discharge to be made. The dreadful label 'bed-blocker' can be avoided in many cases if the NP has pre-planned the discharge with the primary health care team, prior to admission. The result is a far more efficient use of resources and a better deal for patients.

The principle of seeing patients with undiagnosed health problems may be thought to exclude the NP role from inpatient areas. Consider the common situation of an elderly patient with multiple pathology who has been admitted with an acute illness. Pressure on beds is such that they are often discharged in haste and frequently readmitted a few days later, the so-called 'revolving door' syndrome. A thorough NP assessment may facilitate discharge as, although the medical staff have dealt with the acute problem that led to the patient's admission, there may be a range of other subsidiary problems that have not been recognized let alone addressed. The NP assessment may lead to the realization that there are other problems that need action and planning if a successful discharge is to take place and the NP can then work with the primary health care team to ensure a smooth discharge. It may even involve delaying discharge for a day or two but this is worth doing if it prevents a rapid readmission.

The undifferentiated and undiagnosed nature of many of the presenting health problems the NP will encounter are such that extra assessment skills are needed. This includes the ability to carry out a range of physical examination techniques that until now have been thought of as the traditional territory of medicine. The techniques involved (e.g. auscultation, reflex testing, assessing JVP) are straightforward. However, understanding the findings requires knowledge of anatomy, physiology and pathology that goes well beyond what has been taught as part of traditional nursing education. The examination has also to be linked to a structured medical history and diagnostic reasoning process if the NP is to make correct decisions about the likely problems affecting the patient. The technique of taking a structured medical history is also something that NPs need to learn, as they have to incorporate a reasonable working medical diagnosis with their nursing assessment if they are working as the main provider of health care for the patient. The nurse working in an increasingly autonomous role does not have the luxury of leaving the patient's medical problem to the doctors as they simply are not there! Neither can the nurse ignore the medical problems and only concentrate on traditional nursing care.

Perhaps the biggest challenge that NPs and other nurses face when working in increasingly autonomous roles is the challenge of uncertainty. There is no medically made diagnosis or doctor to fall back on. The nurse has to manage the patient's care and make autonomous decisions for which she will be held accountable. Living with uncertainty and making decisions on the balance of probability is not easy and many NPs comment on this as the hardest part of the role.

This discussion on the RCN role definition should by now have made it clear why an honours degree level education is necessary. The NP has to have a strong knowledge base in the biomedical sciences to support newly learnt physical examination techniques and the accountability she carries for increasingly autonomous practice. The skills of medical history taking, diagnostic reasoning and managing uncertainty all have to be learnt in a safe supported environment before the nurses can practice with real patients. Education therefore has to equip the nurse with a toolbox of advanced skills and knowledge which can be applied to a wide range of clinical situations. The NP can be a generalist working for example in primary health care or A&E or she can develop expertise in a specialist area such as orthopaedics or care of the elderly. As we saw in Chapter 5, the legal position is that a nurse carrying out work that previously was undertaken by a doctor is expected to perform to the same standard as a doctor. It is only logical therefore that she has education of the same standard, i.e. honours degree level, to facilitate practice.

Evolutionary perspectives on nursing

Historically, nurses do seem to have a problem with education and change. The introduction of basic education at diploma level has met with much criticism, while the suggestion that pre-registration education should now be raised to degree level arouses strong opposition in many quarters. Nursing remains the only health care occupational group without degree level preparation. It is also the only group aspiring to professional status without degree level education. Nurses have to recognize that the world of health care is moving forward at a rapid rate and education has to keep pace with that change, especially if we are safely to expand nursing horizons in the dramatic ways we now see possible. Advanced nursing roles require advanced nursing education, not a few cheap in house study days put together by the training department.

Nurses cannot practice in new and increasingly autonomous roles if their sole preparation has only been a few medically run study days. The fear of subordinating nursing to medicine is well grounded if medicine controls nursing education. The likely outcome of medical control will not be advanced nurse practitioners but physicians' assistants working closely to medical orders. While the NP role has much to offer patients, other health professionals including doctors, and nurses themselves, it has to be underpinned by appropriate education and national recognition by the statutory body responsible for nursing, the UKCC. With the exception of the RCNI and a small number of universities, this constructive approach is sadly lacking as the UKCC turn their face against the NP and many trusts are unwilling to make the necessary financial investment in NP education.

The reluctance of nursing to embrace expanded nursing roles such as the NP or academic education as a necessary preparation for nursing is symptomatic of nursing's resistance to change. There are many reasons why an institution such as nursing resists change and, as we saw in Chapter 4, culture is one such powerful force. Ford and Walsh (1994) observed that nursing has a problem with change because of the following factors, some of which clearly contribute to this change resistant culture:

❏ The position of nurses as a subordinate group within the health care system which is dominated by doctors and managers

❏ Nursing's historical lack of an objective knowledge base. The absence of evidence-based practice has meant that in the past much nursing has been based upon traditional attitudes and beliefs. Belief systems and their associated attitudes are very stable and change resistant; they are also closely linked with behaviour. The result has been nursing behaviour, i.e. practice, remains difficult to change because it is rooted in subjective human characteristics which are notoriously difficult to change. Evidence however can change as new research findings become available making evidence-based, as opposed to attitude-based, practice more amenable to change
❏ Nurses have traditionally been trained to follow orders rather than educated to think for themselves. There has been a welcome change in the last decade for which pre-registration degree courses and the Diploma in HE must take credit. However, the large majority of nurses are still from the period of nurse training and lack critical appraisal and research utilization skills.

The research which has been carried out on nurses' perceptions of the barriers to changing practice and utilizing research (Walsh, 1997) demonstrates that in the UK the biggest problems are in understanding the research and the lack of authority in the workplace to make change. In the USA where education has been within the academic sector for many years, understanding research is not a major problem, but workplace difficulties and the perception of powerlessness remain the major barriers as in the UK. We will return to the problems of research utilization in the next chapter, however this research does lend support to the views of Ford and Walsh cited above.

There is, however, a more subtle explanation which also contributes to nursing's resistance to change and hence acts to hold back the development of nursing practice. In order to understand this aspect of the problem we have to take a detour into the world of evolutionary biology and explore concepts that were first written about in the UK in relation to nursing by Pediani (1996). Charles Darwin's theory of evolution starts with the observations that in the real world there is variability within organisms and the interaction of organisms with their environment means that some will survive and others will not. Darwin then saw that if whatever helped some organisms to prosper and survive can be passed on to the next generation, then subsequent generations will be better adapted than their parents. Darwin of course did not know about genes and DNA, which we now understand to be the agents responsible for passing information on to subsequent generations. The combination of copying and selection ensures that evolution takes place.

The relevance of this to the problem of nursing and its development becomes apparent when the evolutionary writings of Richard Dawkins are examined. Dawkins (1989) used his analysis of Darwinian evolution to propose a radical new concept, that of the meme. In Dawkins' view, biology is not the only field where evolution is at work. It can also be found in the subjective area of culture and just as the gene is the key to understanding biological evolution so the meme fulfils a similar role in understanding how human culture evolves and changes. Genes are biological replicators, so by analogy, memes are cultural replicators or units of imitation, even though they do not have a physical existence in the same way that genes do. Memes spread by moving from brain to brain and, in order to be successful, they have to have survival value, i.e. be stable and able to penetrate widely through the human 'meme pool'. Memes are therefore ideas that are very stable, widespread and which are successful in being passed from generation to generation just like genes are in biological evolution. Memes are subject to modification as they replicate and only the ones which are best suited to their environment will be successful in replicating themselves from generation to generation (Pediani, 1996). (The ultimate meme in Dawkins' view is God, an idea which has remained stable for a long period and which has survival value because of its psychological appeal in allowing us to make sense of the complex world around us.) These controversial views have relevance to nursing for perhaps nursing has memes of its own which are passed on from generation to generation of nurses without any objective evidence to support them. Perhaps memes are the 'nursing rituals' which Ford and Walsh (1994) first described?

Pediani argues that memes have certain characteristics which will define them, such as fecundity (the extent to which it can spread rapidly through the culture of nursing); longevity (how persistent the idea is); and copying fidelity (how accurately the meme is passed on from one generation of nurses to the next). Good examples of clinical memes are the reluctance of nurse to give opioid analgesia (for fear of inducing drug addiction) and their reluctance to give high concentrations of oxygen via a mask to breathless patients with a history of chronic airways disease (in case it depresses respiratory drive). These two memes have all three characteristics that Pediani identifies; yet the evidence is that patients given good opioid analgesia do not become addicted and patients who are short of breath are far more likely to suffer harm from lack of oxygen than they are from any slight theoretical risk to their respiratory drive.

Humans are unrivalled copiers and memes are therefore readily passed on to subsequent generations. Blackmore (1999) points out that not only are memes replicators but variation is also present as human memory is imperfect; therefore every time we tell a story it changes slightly (the issue of copying fidelity). I am sure you are familiar with how various nursing stories become embellished in the telling! Not all memes are passed on. However, those which are very useful to us, highly memorable or provoke strong reactions are, in Blackmore's view, those which are likely to succeed in making it to the next generation. In other words the conditions for evolution are present: variability, selection and replication.

If memes are ideas, some of which are stable and widespread, effortlessly moving from one generation of nurses to the next, they can be seen as helping to explain nursing's reluctance to change. Evidence and the views of academics and reformers may argue for change but traditional ideas, attitudes and beliefs often block change. Memes, it seems, can triumph over evidence. Other memes have of course failed and faded away, such as nursing models, while others are struggling for survival (dare I suggest primary nursing is one such meme?). Consider now some of the points raised earlier in this chapter in the light of Blackmore's criteria for memetic success.

Let us start with nursing's resistance to academic education and its insistence that nursing is merely about the application of practical common sense with education confined to a few study days to update staff. This is a very useful idea for the experienced nurse who does not possess an academic education and who feels threatened by younger nurses who might acquire greater knowledge via this route. This meme supports her world view and her own self-esteem. The view that nurses should not be expanding their practice by taking on 'doctors work' is very useful again to the nurse who is struggling to keep on top of her current workload. Strong reactions may also be provoked by the suggestion that he or she should take on more work without any extra salary. Unfortunate clashes with one or two doctors may have led to highly memorable critical incidents which result in the nurse not wishing to cooperate with doctors, let alone take on some of their work. All three of Blackmore's criteria are likely to be present for many nurses when the idea of expanding nursing practice at the frontier with medicine is suggested. The result is a meme that is hostile to expansion and wishes to keep nursing well within traditional boundaries. This meme has certainly been evident throughout my nursing career dating back to the early 1970s and is readily passed on under the guise of statements such as 'Nursing is just common sense'; 'Nurses today don't understand basic nursing care'; 'You learn nursing on the wards not in colleges'. Fecundity, longevity and copying fidelity are all strongly present with this particular meme.

The difficulties encountered by nurses wishing to develop care in line with the principles of evidence-based practice may also be viewed in this light. Despite the rhetoric and some examples of good practice, nursing is still by and large reluctant to make patients real partners in care. This is very useful to nurses as it maintains nursing's position of power over patients. One or two highly memorable incidents might also reinforce the view that patients cannot really be trusted to take full responsibility for their care, while a suggestion that flies in the face of over a hundred years of tradition, i.e. the nurse may not know best, is always likely to produce a strong reaction. Blackmore's three criteria for a successful meme of usefulness, a highly memorable incident and evoking a strong reaction are all likely to be present for many nurses. The 'nurse knows best' meme has therefore been successful in spreading through nursing (medicine has the same problem also) and resisting changes which would genuinely give the patient more power. The nursing models meme on the other hand failed to survive and prosper as nursing models were not seen as useful by nurses, failed to produce any memorable incidents and were the subject of supreme indifference by many.

The reader is invited to consider some of the classic nursing rituals, such as getting patients up at 0600 h in the morning, all baths have to be done before lunch, nurse administration of medication on drug rounds and preoperative starving, from the point of view of being nursing memes. They are very useful to nurses in ordering the ward and maintaining power while suggestions of change produces strong reactions. Above all they are copied by each generation of students from the qualified nurses they work with on clinical placement. Learning by imitation was one of the main characteristics of the traditional apprenticeship system of nurse training that existed prior to 1992. It was therefore fertile territory for the transmission of memes as replicators.

The notion that human culture is subject to the laws of evolution, with memes playing the role of genes, may therefore contribute to our understanding of why nursing is so resistant to change. There is an abundance of nursing beliefs that fulfil the role of memes. The conditions for their transmission and replication are highly favourable, especially the reliance in traditional nurse training upon imitation as a means of learning. It is small wonder therefore that developing nursing practice is so difficult. There is, however, a positive side to this suggestion. We wish practice development to result in sustainable changes to practice. If we exploit the ability of successful memes to replicate themselves through successive generations of nurses, this can lead to sustainable change. We therefore need to introduce new ideas (memes) in such a way that they are obviously useful to nurses, memorable and produce an impact which leads to a strong (favourable) reaction. Such a strategy increases the chances of sustainable practice development by ensuring that memes which are newly introduced to the nursing 'meme pool' have a greater chance of being passed on to the next generation. It also emphasizes the importance of the old adage about 'do as I say not as I do', for this approach is counterproductive to meme transmission. Copying and imitation seem to be the key to replication so far as memes are concerned; therefore leaders of change have to lead by example rather than by exhortation. Memes have to be acted out in practice if they are to be replicated.

Biological evolution allows us to shed further light upon nursing's growth and development. Evolution depends heavily upon environment and the ability to adapt. Nightingale faced a very hostile environment in her time but developed a successful strategy for adapting to that environment; she espoused the doctrine of nursing subservience to medicine, which became nursing's first meme. This created a sheltered environment within which nursing could exist and develop. It is only now, a century later, that nursing is showing signs of wanting to move out of this evolutionary niche. This is a measure of how powerful and successful the meme of nursing subservience has been. Its use to nursing was that it allowed it to survive due to the protection and sponsorship of the powerful medical profession, providing nursing knew its place and stayed there.

Dawkins (1989) has suggested that associations of mutual benefit will evolve if each partner can get more out than he puts in. In this case medicine got a great deal more out of the association than it put in. Nurses were loyal hand maidens who ensured the doctors orders were carried out in the early days, and although social norms have changed in the post war years, nurses have still been of enormous benefit to medicine in terms of providing the foundation of patient care needed if the surgeon was to carry out his operative procedures or the physician his complicated therapeutic interventions. Nurses have been the cement and mortar that have held the various bits of the health service together to the advantage of doctors. Doctors have traditionally had a patriarchal view of nursing and some can still be heard to refer to 'my nurses'. What has medicine put back? This patriarchy has, on occasion, protected nurses from outside hostile forces, undoubtedly contributed to the education of nurses (though with medical ideas) and has given nursing support and a sense of confidence, though not in itself. Nursing in the early days was able to establish itself and survive as a respectable profession. This may well be seen as nursing getting more out than it put into the relationship, especially given Victorian ideas about duty, servitude and a woman's role which would see as normal much of what we would see as oppression. The nursing/medical association can be seen as growing out of this evolutionary principle and being passed on as a meme from one generation of nurses to the next.

It is only in the last 20 years or so that this has begun to change. The reason for this change can be found in the changes that are occurring in the environment, both within health care and society in general. Nursing has matured to a position where its leaders consider they get far less out of this association than they put in. Nursing subservience is a price not worth paying for medical patronage; consequently the old association is breaking down as nurses seek to move away from this evolutionary niche. Changes in nursing education mean that student nurses are less reliant upon simply copying the behaviour of qualified staff (the subservience meme). They now read research and discuss the nature of relationships with other professional groups. These are unfavourable conditions for the replication of the subservience meme! It is not surprising therefore that nurses now seek a position of partnership with doctors and are developing new adaptive strategies to survive in the changing world of health care.

Perhaps nurse practitioners are looking to form a new association with medicine based upon the same principle that we each get more out than we put in, but in a different kind of relationship. The NP puts a lot of effort into education and develops her NP role to be complementary to the doctors and in return is allowed much greater autonomy and, as a result, greater job satisfaction. The doctor puts effort into helping to train and educate the NP and also has to invest time in developing the role, but the return is that the work undertaken by the NP reduces the pressures and strains on the doctor. The NP frequently takes on aspects of patient care that medical training does not equip doctors for or which they simply do not find interesting or challenging. They are therefore relieved to have a NP take over these aspects of care knowing that the NP will refer the patient to the doctor if his or her medical skills are needed. Both NP and doctor can therefore set up a mutual association which allows each to get out more than they put in, leading to the evolution of a successful relationship which will be likely to last, providing it is not subject to any major environmental changes. Such changes will require the association to adapt and restore the mutual back-scratching relationship if it is to survive.

Summary

This chapter has explored the development of nursing at its boundary with medicine. The principles and ideas suggested here are equally applicable at other boundaries such as those with radiography, midwifery, the rehabilitative therapies or social work. By looking beyond the boundaries of nursing and traditional health disciplines we can see that there are powerful explanations for some of the apparent difficulties that are associated with boundary conditions. We should not be surprised to find such challenges lying in wait at the boundaries of nursing, it is only to be expected when nursing is considered as part of the real world state of things or placed in its wider context. Instead of trying to impose artificial boundaries and censuring those who straddle these frontiers, we should be applauding and supporting such nurses for taking nursing practice forward into new areas. Perhaps what happens out there is hybrid practice but that is only to be expected in the real world where boundaries are all fractal fuzz and straight lines are conspicuous by their absence. Evolution theory holds vital clues to understanding how nursing has got to where it is today and consequently where it might be heading tomorrow. We should exploit insights such as meme theory in the cause of practice development.

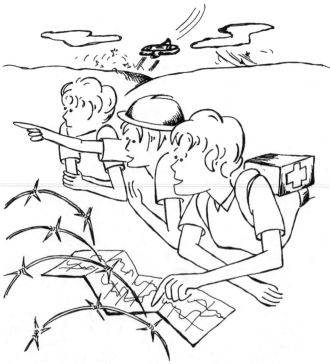

DEVELOPING NURSING PRACTICE CAN FEEL LIKE A REAL BATTLE

References

Blackmore, S. (1999). Meme, myself, I. *New Scientist*, 13 March, 40–44.

Castledine, G. (1995). Defining specialist nursing. *British Journal of Nursing*, **4**, 5, 264–265.

Cohen, J. and Stewart, I. (1994). *The Collapse of Chaos*. London: Penguin.

Coveney, P. and Highfield, R. (1995). *Frontiers of Complexity; The Search for Order in a Chaotic World*. New York: Faber and Faber.

Dawkins, R. (1989). *The Selfish Gene* (2nd edn). Oxford: Oxford University Press.

Edwards, B., Holloway, I., Galvin, K., Andrews, C. and Potter, P. (1999). Nurse Practitioners; are we being true to the spirit of nursing? *Emergency Nurse*, **7**, 3, 26–31.

Ford, P. and Walsh, M. (1994). *New Rituals for Old*. Oxford: Butterworth-Heinemann.

Giroux, H. (1985). Introduction. In: Freire, P. (ed.) *The Politics of Education*. New York: Macmillan.

MacAlister, L. and Chiam, M. (1995). Why do nurses agree to take on doctors' roles. *British Journal of Nursing*, **4**, 21, 1238–1239.

Meek, S., Kendall, J., Porter, J. and Freij, R. (1998). Can acident and emergency nurse practitioners interpret radiographs? A multicentre study. *Journal of Accident and Emergency Medicine*, **15**, 2, 105–107.

Parnell, C. S. (1885). Speech at an Election Rally, Cork.

Pediani, R. (1996). Chaos and evolution in nursing research. *Journal of Advanced Nursing*, **23**, 645–646.

Ray, M. (1998). Complexity and nursing science. *Nursing Science Quarterly*, **11**, 3, 91–93.

Senior, K. (1999). ENP scheme: highlighting the barriers. *Emergency Nurse*, **6**, 9, 28–32.

UKCC (1992). *Code of Professional Conduct*. London: UKCC.

UKCC (1994). *Standards for Post-registration Education and Practice*. London: UKCC.

Royal College of Nursing (1996). *Council Position Statement on the Role of the Nurse Practitioner*. London: RCN.

Walsh, M. (1997). How nurses perceive barriers to research implementation. *Nursing Standard*, **11**, 29, 34–39.

Walsh, M. (1999). Nurses and nurse practitioners; priorities in care. *Nursing Standard*, **13**, 24, 38–42.

CHAPTER 8

Practice development

There was never any more inception than there is
  now,
Nor any more youth or age than there is now,
And will never be any more perfection than
  there is now,
Nor any more heaven or hell than there is now.

Walt Whitman (1855) Song of Myself.

Introduction

How often do you hear nurses of a certain age harking back to the 'good
old days' of starched aprons and caps, students who knew their place
(usually making beds) and proper training rather than this so-called
education, that stops students learning proper basic nursing skills?
Dwelling on nostalgia is one way of escaping from the harsh realities of
today and nursing is by no means unusual in harking back to a mythical
golden age when all things were better than they are today. This of course
is Walt Whitman's point in the quotation at the start of this chapter. The
opening lines of this poem are also worth quoting as they express the
feelings that lie behind the transmission of nursing tradition:

I celebrate myself and sing myself.
And what I assume you shall assume

In this way traditional nursing proclaims itself, making it clear that
students will work to the same assumptions (memes) that have guided
generations of nurses. However, in this age of change, individual
accountability and evidence-based practice, assumptions and traditions
are of less and less value. If nursing is to keep pace with the times and
fulfil its fundamental mission of placing the patient's welfare first, then
practice has to develop and move on. The first step in practice
development is to stop looking backwards to the good old days,
recognize that things have improved and can continue to improve into
the future. Assumptions and rituals are not however a sound base for

practice development. Binoculars rather than rose-coloured spectacles are needed to scan the horizon for exciting opportunities and ideas which will allow us to take nursing forward.

Practice development: from NDU to PDU

The pathway followed by practice development during the 1990s can be summarized by the strange initials above. The decade began with the nursing development unit (NDU) concept but has ended with some radically new insights summarized by the mathematical formula SI = f(E,C,F). Non-mathematicians should read on as this formula is merely a way of summarizing the relationship between successful implementation (SI) of change and the three important contributory factors of evidence (E), context (C) and facilitation (F). But first, let us deal with the more familiar NDU concept, which was hailed as providing a major opportunity for the development of nursing practice.

Nursing Development Units had their origins in the 1980s with the pioneering work of Alan Pearson (Burford), Steve Wright (Tameside) and Sue Pembrey (Oxford). The common theme that united these three was a desire to establish an environment in which nursing could develop, new ideas could be tried and which would act as a showcase for the value of nursing. The NDU would therefore demonstrate the therapeutic potential of nursing in a proactive way rather than seeing nursing as something passive which followed the prescriptions and orders of others (Page *et al.*, 1998). By the start of the 1990s the Kings Fund had taken the NDU concept on board and allocated £500 000 to prime the setting up of a series of NDUs. This network grew further with the Department of Health making £3.2 million available to establish a total of 30 such units. This movement offered nursing an opportunity to show that it could make a difference to health care.

The thinking that defined the NDU movement has been summarized by Page *et al.* (1998) as follows:

❑ Maximizing the involvement of patients as partners in care
❑ Empowerment of individual nurses who in turn take on more autonomy
❑ Creating a change friendly environment committed to research-based care
❑ Collective development of high quality care and sharing new ideas
❑ Evaluation of the effectiveness and efficiency of practice.

Few would disagree with these goals. However, the NDU movement has found the going difficult. The 1990s have seen further NDUs come into being but, at the same time, others have fallen by the wayside. The NDU movement has been swimming against the tide for much of the decade as the climate in the NHS for most of 1990s has been against empowerment, sharing and a sense of collective cooperation. The 1990s was the decade of macho management, the internal market, competition and cutting back of resources by the Conservative government responsible for this market culture. This emphasizes the importance of culture in determining the success of any enterprise within an organization (see Chapter 1) as clearly the NDU culture was at odds with the prevailing NHS culture of the internal market.

Each NDU was set up with a clinical leader whose role was pivotal to success. Research by Christian and Norman (1998) has shown, however, that the clinical leaders in these units have faced many problems. A major dilemma was the conflict created by being both a manager with responsibility for an NDU and therefore for implementing change and being a clinical leader who had to persuade more senior managers to let change occur. NDU leaders became very frustrated when their immediate managers did not support the change agenda and the unit suffered as a result. The other major problem encountered by leaders was lack of ownership, particularly among the more junior staff. This seems paradoxical as the NDU philosophy was all about empowerment of staff. Clearly this is something easier said than done and suggests that there are forces at work which act to prevent junior staff becoming involved, even when the leader wants them to. These two findings suggest that NDU clinical leaders struggled because of problems in facilitating change and environmental factors.

Further research into the NDU network by Redfearn and Stevens (1998) found that the promotion of needs led, individualized care, practised in partnership with patients could be recognized in the mission statements prepared by most of the units. The other two most common aims were the promotion of excellence in practice and staff support/supervision which were each reported by just over half the NDUs surveyed. These aims fit with the key points listed by Page *et al.* above with one notable exception, evaluation of the impact of the NDU on patient care. Wright and Salvage (1995), two of the early NDU pioneers, have repeatedly stressed the importance of evaluation yet, unfortunately, it does not seem to have taken place. This issue was brought to a head when a Department of Health funded research project into the effectiveness of NDUs was abandoned as insufficient evidence had been gathered to allow the researchers to investigate the question. This embarrassing state of affairs was reported in Nursing Standard (1998) with one of the researchers, Professor Sally Redfearn quoted as saying 'We don't know if the units were any good for patients'.

The NDU movement was set up to show the value of nursing to patient care and some 10 years later, a major research project aimed at investigating this question had to be abandoned for lack of evidence. We are therefore lacking the convincing evidence that might show whether NDUs make any difference to patient outcomes. This is an unfortunate blow to the credibility of NDUs and nursing as a whole.

The work on NDUs has inspired Australian nurses to establish Clinical Development Units (Nursing). Greenwood (1999) has reported on a network of nine such units established in 1997 around Sydney. The aim is to set up nurse led, multidisciplinary, practice development units which explains the abbreviation CDU(N). Preparation of clinical leaders is seen as crucial and each person receives six blocks of 2 days' training in readiness for taking on the role. These units share the NDU goal of allowing nursing to demonstrate its therapeutic value. However, Greenwood stresses this has to be in a multidisciplinary environment. The CDU(N) projects are not seen as flagships or elitist by their proponents but, rather, are concerned with standards and projects that all areas can and should aspire towards. Greenwood argues these two key points concerning multidisciplinary working and a non-elitist approach differentiate the CDU(N) from the original British NDU movement. Although these units have been acclaimed as a success, Greenwood's paper cannot produce any evidence to show they have had an impact upon patient outcomes. Until such evidence is forthcoming, the CDU(N) remains in the same category as the NDU, a worthwhile project aimed at raising the profile of nursing but of no demonstrable value to the patient.

The multidisciplinary theme introduced by the Australians has, however, been developed further in the UK. An alternative approach to practice development has been proposed which is critical of the NDUs concentration on nursing alone. Page *et al.* (1998) argue that practice should be driven by patient need not professional aspirations. This different approach therefore favours a multidisciplinary style of development leading to Practice Development Units (PDU) being established with many of the same aspirations of the original NDUs. The difference is that these are seen in terms of teamworking across professions. To focus on one profession only in what is in reality a multiprofessional environment is seen as inappropriate and undermining good teamwork by advocates of the PDU approach. In fairness to the NDU approach, it has to be seen in its historical context. In the early 1980s the profile of nursing was considerably lower than it is today and therefore an attempt to raise that profile via the NDU movement was justifiable. However, time has moved on and throughout this book I have argued the need for nursing to expand its scope of practice but, in the process, to recognize this will impact upon a range of other professions. Negotiations about the boundaries of practice with other groups of staff are essential. To succeed, such negotiations need mutual understanding and trust. Nursing therefore has to look outward not inward. Some 15 years on from the early NDU work, it is now time to work on multiprofessional practice development. This is a sign of the growing self-confidence and maturity of nursing.

The PDU movement also places great emphasis upon research and evaluation of practice development, as did the proponents of NDUs. If the proponents of the PDUs can be more successful than NDUs in carrying out this research, they would be in a stronger position to argue their cause. Reliable evidence of real improvements in patient outcomes (clinical effectiveness) is worth its weight in gold.

The PDU has another similarity with the NDU in that it is located on a single clinical area (ward, department, health centre or unit). The need for peer group support has been recognized and led to the setting up of networks for this to happen. One such project networked 13 PDUs in a single NHS English Region (based on Oxford) and has been studied by Ward *et al.* (1998) over a 12-month period. PDU leaders met monthly and their meetings were facilitated by staff from the Royal College of Nursing Institute in Oxford. Evaluation of change was highlighted in these meetings, marking a move on from the NDU approach. This study identified the following key problems faced by these PDUs:

- ❏ Few of the project leaders were properly prepared for being change agents
- ❏ Lack of managerial support caused problems for which PDU leaders were unprepared
- ❏ Trusts failed to own the PDUs
- ❏ Project leaders lacked knowledge of research and development techniques and skills
- ❏ Communication difficulties existed between the different projects and between PDU leaders and their supervisors. This was mainly caused by geographical problems of distance.

Despite these problems a great deal of positive staff development work had gone on although, as with the NDUs, there is a paucity of reported patient outcome data supporting the effectiveness of the PDU concept. If PDUs help to foster better interprofessional relationships, they could make a major contribution to advancing clinical practice for all professions, including nursing. This is because the boundaries of practice are the most fertile areas for practice development and, as we argued in the preceding chapter, professional groups have to cooperate and share territory in these grey areas rather than fight each other over imaginary and artificial dividing lines which do not exist in the real world.

One common theme that links both NDUs and PDUs is that they are isolated within a Trust. It is usual also to seek *external* accreditation by an outside body. Dissemination of good practice lies at the heart of the rationale for the existence of PDU/NDUs yet the policy of locating all practice development work in a single identified unit merely interferes with dissemination. This is compounded by the perceptions of elitism that inevitably arises in such a situation. It also sends a message to the rest of the Trust that we do not think you can develop practice. Such a message may or may not be intended but that is how it will be received by many staff. It is a waste of resources not to involve all staff in practice development, which can be the effect of having a single dedicated PDU/ NDU. The interaction of staff from different parts of the Trust can be very creative in an unpredictable way, however this cannot happen in a single unit approach. The principle of full staff involvement and a grassroots approach to change indicates that a PDU will only succeed if all staff are involved rather than it being the pet project of a single manager who initiated the project.

Consideration of these points suggests that the PDU approach might work best in a self-contained unit such as a community hospital, a mental health unit area such as a medium secure unit or with a primary health care team in a defined geographical area. However, within a general hospital setting there may be problems if a single surgical or medical ward is selected for example. One of the most publicized successful PDUs is the one at Seacroft Hospital in Yorkshire and this actually consists of four wards comprising the elderly/medical care department, again emphasizing the importance of networking staff together rather than going it alone on a single ward.

Outside accreditation can also have a negative effect in that it conveys a message that we, within the Trust, are not good enough to recognize good practice when we see it. Internal clinical audit still has a long way to go to achieve widespread acceptance, so outsiders scrutinizing and challenging practice may feel very threatening. Accreditation can become a very bureaucratic process involving a great deal of time and expense, leaving staff asking whether it is seriously worth it. It also places a great deal of pressure on staff. The accreditation process can become a paper exercise in which a great deal of effort goes into producing paper evidence that the unit meets the criteria of the accrediting body. In the process, the work of actually developing practice can become of secondary importance, which rather defeats the aim of the exercise. It may well be that the perceived value of external accreditation was partially derived from the pernicious effects of the internal market. Having a 'kite marked' PDU could be seen as enhancing the prestige of a Trust and therefore its position in the market place when competing for contracts to provide care.

Page *et al.* (1998) consider one of the main advantages of the PDU approach is the flexibility and adaptability it generates. They feel that the NDU was defined in concrete terms too soon and became a victim of its own high profile. As a result it was unable to adapt to the rapidly changing and hostile environment of the 1990s. The PDU is described as being a more adaptable creature and Page *et al.* openly admit that the Seacroft Unit fell upon hard times after its successful first 2 years of operation. This was due to major upheavals and uncertainty created by NHS reorganization which, in turn, led to key staff members leaving. Resources were also squeezed hard which had a detrimental effect so that for a while the PDU was almost moribund. However, the Seacroft PDU was described as a flexible, dynamic, model which allowed it to survive and adapt, especially as new staff shared the vision and view of the way forward with existing staff. Page *et al.* consider this shared vision fundamental to success along with the need for expert facilitation and listening skills if a truly empowered workforce is to develop.

There are two striking features of the analysis offered by Page *et al.* which explain why their PDU has been successful. First is their use of evolutionary language as they frequently talk of their PDU surviving and adapting, the need for adaptability in such a changing environment, and the suggestion that NDUs have not lived up to their early promise because they were unable to adapt. However, in the preceding chapter I suggested that there were powerful analogies in evolutionary theory for nursing development. Without directly referring to evolution, Page *et al.* continually use its language. The other feature of their account is the importance of the context within which practice development was occurring and the value of facilitation. These are issues that will be expanded upon later in this chapter when the practice development model of Kitson *et al.* (1998) is explored, as context and facilitation are crucial to their model.

Networking

The PDU approach therefore can be seen as a welcome evolution from the NDU idea or meme, but it still has significant problems so long as it is located in one single area. Perhaps the next evolutionary step is to network the PDU throughout the Trust? Greenwood (1999) for example describes how the Australian CDU(N) movement, described earlier, is concentrating on networking its leaders together. There is an obvious biological analogy here as, of course, one of the major landmarks in the evolution of life was when single cell organisms evolved into multi-cellular animals which could achieve far more by networking their individual cells into a coordinated animal. We have already argued in the preceding chapter that an organization is far more than the sum of its constituent parts and networking throughout a trust could allow practice development to appear as an emergent property (p. 112).

This networking approach has been developed by Steve Wright and the author in Cumbria. The key people in making any hospital function are the clinical specialists and ward sister/charge nurse grades, for they are the clinical leaders. We have developed a practice development networking approach which concentrates upon these members of staff and after working this through with three separate acute trusts we suggest the following steps might be followed:

❑ Convene a meeting of these staff. Open the meeting with senior management (e.g. chief nurse and chief executive) making a strong commitment to practice development. This sends a clear message to staff that they do have the backing of top management and helps break down the 'them and us' barriers that so bedevil the NHS at present. The 'them and us' theme will require a great deal of effort to work through, during the project. We have found breaking down this mind set to be an essential part of the empowerment process. It is easy for staff to slip into a state of learned helplessness and assume that they will never be allowed to develop practice while blaming 'them', i.e. management, for this state of affairs. Claiming back responsibility for your own practice is a necessary precursor for accountability and clinical governance

❑ After senior management have withdrawn from the meeting, we act as empathic outsiders, to facilitate an open discussion about the problems facing clinical staff and the barriers preventing practice development. At this very early stage, it is better if management have withdrawn but they will be reintroduced to the group later. There is an element of catharsis involved here as staff have an opportunity to express their frustrations and disappointments. It is important to know when to stop this process before it becomes too negative and destructive and begin to turn things to a more positive direction

❑ We aim to conclude the initial meeting by getting staff to identify a series of topics they want to know more about

❏ The staff then attend a series of workshop days at monthly intervals. The first workshop concentrates on team building. The increasing fragmentation and pressure of work in hospitals makes it harder for staff actually to know each other, therefore team building work is absolutely necessary and best done away from the hospital or education centre. A programme of workshop days follows at monthly intervals covering topics that the staff have chosen for themselves. The time off the wards also helps demonstrate the commitment of senior management to supporting practice development

❏ At the end of 6–9 months the key clinical leaders have started to become a knowledgeable team and are now ready to tackle practice development. They are now ready to meet the Chief Nurse and discuss how they want to develop practice. Obviously the Trust has a say in this process as, together with the patients, they are one of the main stakeholders.

❏ Each member of staff is the leader for a project in their own area which we facilitate as outsiders. We find this means that change is owned by staff and perceived as useful to clinical practice. A key part of this stage is identifying measures that can show whether the change is making a difference to patient care and outcomes. This work is currently underway

❏ Staff continue to meet as a learning set at quarterly intervals to give each other mutual support. In the future a second wave of staff can be brought into a similar scheme with the first group acting as practice development mentors. We have not reached this stage with our work yet.

NHS trusts have a substantial number of units or vouchers, allocated by the Continuing Education Consortia, which they can trade in with their local higher education provider to pay for continuing professional development. Normally, they purchase courses with these vouchers. An alternative way forward might be to convert these vouchers into education staff time made available to work with clinical staff as facilitators to develop practice in the way suggested here. If trusts purchased a mix of taught courses and practice development facilitation, rather than just courses, they might find they got better value for money in terms of *developing practice*.

The SI = f(E,C,F) model

The model described above has evolved as a result of past experience, local circumstances and reading the literature on practice development. This evolution has taken place at the same time as a great deal of work has been undertaken on practice development by Alison Kitson and her colleagues in the RCN Institute at Oxford. Our approach is congruent with Kitson's work which is enshrined in the SI=f(E,C,F) formula that introduced this section.

Kitson *et al.* (1998) propose that the successful implementation of practice development is a function of (i.e. depends upon) the evidence base (E), the context within which change is to occur (C) and the degree of facilitation (F). Their model arose from a rejection of the linear model of practice development as too simple. By a linear model they mean the simple steps of accessing the research evidence, disseminating it via education and conferences in order that it may then be implemented and finally evaluating how effective it has been. Kitson *et al.* rightly point out this model has had little success in changing practice and a more sophisticated approach is needed.

A moment's reflection suggests there are many other factors that influence the uptake of new ideas and these factors are all at work simultaneously. This model proposes capturing these factors in the three variables of evidence, context and facilitation. Each of these variables may be assigned a value ranging from strong to weak. If all three are strong, successful implementation is highly likely but if they are all weak, then it is unlikely. These are the extreme conditions and in between there is a very complex range of possibilities. One particular combination that nurses will be familiar with might be where there is a strong evidence base for changing practice but the context and facilitation are weak, resulting in much frustration but little change. However, the model suggests that problems caused by an unfavourable context can be at least partially overcome by strong evidence and good facilitation.

In order to get to grips with this model, we need to look at it in more detail. Evidence consists of three main sources of which research is only one. Alongside research we should also place professional judgement (based upon critical reflection) and patient preferences as equally valid sources of evidence. Strong research evidence is derived from rigorous, methodologically sound, systematic evaluations and may be either qualitative or quantitative. Critical appraisal skills are necessary to separate such research from poor quality work which has flaws in its methods, or is unsystematic, being little better than anecdotal description.

A forum such as a consensus conference or a detailed literature review may show strong agreement of professional opinion on a topic. This can give rise to a strong evidence base derived from professional judgement about what is effective in improving patient care. However, if professional opinion is totally divided about an issue or if the opinions of only a small number are sought, this is clearly weak evidence about effectiveness. The view of a single ward sister or consultant does not constitute strong evidence from a professional judgement perspective. Much nursing care in the past has however had this kind of evidence base, the attitudes and beliefs of a single powerful individual amounting at times to little more than personal prejudice.

Effective clinical supervision networks can greatly help the nurse reflect critically upon practice in a safe non-judgemental environment. It is the critical reflection that transforms experience into evidence and learning, however, and this is a skill that has to be learnt. Nurses who are developing new roles may find it hard to locate peers with whom they can conduct clinical supervision sessions. Two solutions which we have implemented locally involve the use of video-conference technology and case presentations. The former involves linking three sites in Cumbria, where geography is a problem, using video-conferencing technology which allows nurses to conduct supervision meetings with their peers many miles away with complete confidentiality. There is no reason why nurses in Belfast and Bognor Regis or Aberdeen and Abergavenny cannot exploit this technology for clinical supervision. We have also found that our nurse practitioner graduates enjoy meeting every month in the evening with two of the group taking it in turn to bring along some interesting and difficult cases to present to the group for discussion. Meetings are facilitated by teaching staff and last well into the night as a whole range of fascinating issues are debated. In this way individual practitioners reflect critically upon real practice issues and learn from their clinical experience. Processes such as these help nurses develop critical judgement skills about their practice and build a sound professional consensus about the effectiveness of care. This is professional practice development. It is a million light years away from nursing's tradition of just doing what you were told by the figure in authority which leads to the 'my assumptions are your assumptions' position described in the introduction.

The views of patients constitute a third source of evidence. The importance of this perspective was identified by Ovretveit (1992) who analyses quality into three components: professional, managerial and client centred. The professional component is that which we as nurses consider makes good care and therefore consists of a mixture of research and professional judgement, while the managerial component is about cost effective uses of resources. Using patient satisfaction with care as evidence therefore has a common sense appeal to it, sounds ethically correct and is derived from the work of respected experts on health care quality such as Ovretveit. It is not so simple, however, as French (1981) observed two decades ago that patient satisfaction surveys produce uniformly high scores which are unable to discriminate between different standards of care. McColl et al. (1996) consider this to be still the case hence their work on developing the Newcastle Satisfaction with Nursing Scales (NSNS) as a discriminatory tool that can produce reliable evidence about the quality of care as seen from the patients' perspective.

There are several problems with simply asking patients to tick a box to show their satisfaction with care. Patients may give socially desirable answers as they do not want to upset the staff or, if they are still patients at the time, they might be worried about the consequences of appearing critical or even ungrateful. Modern health care is a very complex process involving many different staff and services. A single rating cannot capture the complexity of the situation where nurses are very caring, the food awful, the doctors do their best but are always too busy, the ward runs out of bed linen at the weekend and you were left waiting on a trolley outside X-ray for over an hour because no porter was available! The NSNS tool is an attempt to get around this problem by just focusing on nursing. Other problems stem from the fact that most patients are elderly and as Thomas et al. (1996) point out, the elderly are more deferential and less likely to complain, especially as they remember life before the NHS. This introduces systematic bias into any attempt to measure satisfaction as part of the evidence base.

Despite these problems, the views of patients are a crucial part of the evidence base. The challenge is to discover reliable ways of finding out what patients really think of the care they received and crucially of the sort of care they would like in the future. The strength of patient preferences as a source of evidence can be nil, i.e. nobody has asked the patients what they think or very weak if a methodologically flawed and simplistic tick box approach is used. Alternatively a well carried out survey with a reliable and valid tool such as the NSNS or individual interviews can generate strong evidence of patient preferences.

Practice development therefore needs the strongest possible evidence base and this must include staff education to allow them to access good, up to date research. This also requires libraries to be readily available to staff, which has become an increasing problem in the 1990s as colleges of nursing have been closed and educational resources have been centralized on to a small number of university sites. Staff cannot be expected to implement evidence-based practice without access to the evidence. It is also unrealistic to expect staff to develop practice if they are denied access to education. Access to education is a crucial element in building the evidence base for change, but on its own is not enough.

It is necessary to repeat that evidence consists of multiple sources other than empirical research. The randomized controlled trial (RCT) is the best method of determining effectiveness (i.e. answering questions of cause and effect), however, Clarke (1999) reminds us that one form of evidence should not dominate others and that nursing has a responsibility to contribute to that evidence. The danger of course is that the power of the medical profession may lead to the domination of empirical evidence, particularly the RCT, at the expense of many other equally valid sources of evidence. Nurses involved in practice development must beware of this danger and be prepared to argue for the validity of other sources of evidence besides the RCT. A further point made by Clarke concerns the nurse's own prejudices and value systems. They should not be allowed to cloud the evidence and introduce bias. A fear of maths should not be grounds for rejecting empirical data as evidence, while strong concern for the patient's point of view has to be balanced with a recognition of the value of objective data gathered by neutral researchers.

If evidence is a necessary but not sufficient condition for change, we also have to look at the role of context and facilitation. The context can be favourable to practice development (strong) or unfavourable (weak). Staff relationships and the culture of the area are crucial ingredients of context. If staff are valued and empowered, encouraged to suggest new ideas and attend courses and above all work within a democratic, change friendly culture, there is a strong context for practice development. Good management skills and strong clinical leadership also contribute towards a favourable context. The final ingredient is measurement of progress. This involves both regular, constructive staff appraisal and also clinical audit. In this way the performance of staff can be measured both as individuals and from the perspective of patient outcomes. The implementation of clinical supervision and clinical governance will assist in creating the right context for development as they both support and empower clinical staff.

Kitson *et al.* cite examples of the role of context in helping or hindering practice development. A revealing example is reported by Tinkler *et al.* (1999) who set about implementing evidence-based clinical guidelines in the field of leg ulcer management.

Tinkler *et al.* (1999) were working without the benefit of reliable research to help them devise an implementation strategy. They set about introducing two effective compression bandaging regimens which had a strong evidence base to support them. The project was based in the community. Although the authors report that they succeeded in a significant number of their goals, they describe the major barriers to progress as follows:

❑ General practitioners refused to allow 'their' nursing staff (e.g. practice nurses) to treat patients in the community (with the new bandaging regimen) who were not on their lists
❑ When patients were hospitalized for whatever reason, the bandaging regimen was not followed by hospital staff as they had not been able to attend training sessions organized for community staff to teach the correct procedure
❑ Some components of the bandaging system were not available on prescription and extra funding had to be obtained from the Health Authority to allow the project to proceed.

The first two of these barriers to practice development are clearly related to contextual difficulties. The medical culture of patient ownership and the traditional divide between hospital and primary health care probably contributed much to the difficulties experienced by Tinkler and her colleagues. In reflecting on the project they comment how involvement of senior nurses in the hospital and the hospital tissue viability nurse might have resulted in more involvement of hospital staff in the training programme and consequently patients would have been able to continue their bandaging regimen when admitted to hospital for whatever reason.

Facilitation is defined by Kitson *et al.* as the technique of making things easier for others. A facilitator can be an outsider (as in the model outlined above) or an insider. Either way a facilitator should not be confused with an opinion leader but it is helpful if the facilitator identifies opinion leaders and works with them. Strong facilitation involves a person who brings the qualities of approachability, openness, supportiveness, self-confidence and creative thinking to the role. He or she should also be able to work across boundaries as a multidisciplinary approach greatly assists practice development. The role of the facilitator also needs to be understood by all concerned and not confused with that of the clinical leader responsible for the clinical practice of the area under development.

The evidence-based practice movement is generating clinical guide-lines to guide practitioners. Such guidelines consist of statements that will help nurses make decisions about the best course of action to follow in given circumstances. They are therefore a key source of evidence for practice. Thomas (1999) has reviewed the topic of guidelines and suggests there is evidence to indicate they can change nursing practice and improve patient outcomes. However, as she points out, clinical guidelines alone will change little unless they are accompanied by an implementation strategy. The problem is neatly summed up by Newman *et al.* (1998) who state that interventions which focus on the skills and knowledge of nurses alone without looking at how such skills and knowledge may be implemented are unlikely to be successful in changing practice.

Unfortunately, as Cheater and Closs (1997) have observed there is a dearth of research into the best methods of implementing clinical guidelines for nurses. Some work has been done in medicine but it is dangerous to assume that what works in medicine will automatically work in nursing. This is a point we will come back to later in the next chapter. Suffice it to say that based upon medical research, Cheater and Closs remind us that there are key questions to ask in implementing clinical guidelines:

- ❑ Are we clear whom the guidelines are targeted on and how can we ensure they will reach this audience?
- ❑ In what form should guidelines be published and disseminated?
- ❑ How do we monitor and evaluate the implementation of the guidelines and their subsequent effectiveness?
- ❑ How much will this all cost?

Thomas urges nurses to be involved in the development of guidelines (rather than be passive recipients) as this is likely to increase a sense of ownership and hence generate a more positive attitude. If nurses develop their own guidelines they also need the critical appraisal skills to allow them to reject poor quality research and also work that fails convincingly to show the effectiveness of practice. Nurses must avoid the unthinking implementation of guidelines produced elsewhere. Such a 'recipe book' approach is fraught with danger as ineffective procedures can become cloaked in the false respectability of 'evidence'. Thomas goes on to emphasize the importance of recognizing barriers to change and factors which will promote the facilitation of change within any implementation strategy. Context and facilitation are therefore placed alongside evidence as essential ingredients of practice development.

Clinical guidelines do allow the nurse to accept more accountability for his or her practice with an easier conscience. The knowledge that the procedure you are following is based upon experts reviewing a substantial body of evidence and publishing it as best practice should give you the confidence that helps you become an accountable practitioner. It also strengthens your position in regard of any legal problems that may arise from a claim for negligence (Chapter 5). However, it does create a certain tension over autonomy and merely emphasizes the relative nature of that concept as it may be argued that strict adherence to clinical guidelines removes a practitioner's autonomy. Guidelines do not exempt the nurse from having the responsibility of making clinical decisions for which he or she is accountable. The key decision is whether the patient is suitable for the guidelines, as implementing a clinical guideline on an inappropriate patient could be argued to be negligent. It is in making the decision not to implement a guideline that professional judgement is needed. Justifying and, if necessary, defending that decision involve truly accountable practice. Nurses should not be slaves to clinical guidelines or else they will become the rituals of tomorrow but rather use them as a starting point to plan patient care. The guidelines will probably be appropriate for the large majority of patients, but not all, and the skill or artistry of nursing is to recognize the patient who requires a different approach.

Reflection on the literature concerning the NDU/PDU movement demonstrates the importance of context and facilitation. The NDU/PDU clinical leaders' reported sense of isolation and being unprepared for the pressures of acting as change agents underlines the importance of facilitation. Problems caused by lack of management support and lack of ownership by junior staff were apparent. These findings are consistent with investigations of barriers to research utilization carried out by Funk and Champagne (1991). This research was carried out in North America but Walsh (1997) has replicated the study in the UK with a sample of hospital and community nurses. Both pieces of research showed that workplace barriers such as others not allowing the nurse to implement change, the nurse feeling he or she had insufficient authority to change practice or the workplace was just too busy were the prime barriers. There was no statistically significant difference in the perceptions of hospital or community nurses in this respect.

There was however a significant difference between the North American and British nurses when the issue of understanding the research evidence was explored. This was not seen as a major barrier by the North Americans but it was by the British nurses. In fact of the 27 items in the Funk and Champagne Barriers tool, understanding statistical evidence was rated as the single biggest barrier in the UK. This is particularly significant in light of the warning that nurses cannot be selective in choosing the evidence upon which to base practice (Clark, 1999). This finding suggests that much empirical evidence may go unheeded or be accepted uncritically because nurses lack the skills to understand the statistical methods used.

If British nurses report that understanding the research evidence is a major barrier to research utilization, this has major implications. It reinforces the need for better education of nurses in the UK. It is difficult to see how we can aspire to professional status or expand nursing practice if we cannot read and understand research evidence. Comparison with nurse education in North America leads to the obvious conclusion that a university degree based educational system has produced nurses who can understand research evidence more readily than their British counterparts. Whatever reforms in nursing education may be planned in the next few years, a continued failure to equip nurses with the academic skills associated with degree level education will only hinder the development of practice. The problems caused by struggling to understand research findings also supports the Kitson *et al.* model for practice development with its emphasis upon evidence as one of the three pillars upon which practice development is built.

Summary

This chapter has briefly reviewed the recent history of organizational strategies aimed at developing nursing practice. The NDU movement has struggled as it was swimming against the ideological tide for much of the last decade and it is now increasingly giving way to a more multi-professional approach. NDUs were successful in raising awareness and even just by linking the two words 'nursing' and 'development' in the same phrase made a major political point. Nursing could and should be developed, and nurses were the best people to do it. The importance of that message cannot be underestimated. The value of networking practice development work has been emphasized rather than leaving it in single isolated units. This is especially important in view of the more philosophical discussion of notions of complexity in the preceding chapter; the whole is greater than the sum of its individual parts. The chapter concludes with the view that evidence is a necessary but not sufficient condition for practice development. It is essential to recognize the interplay of context and facilitation with evidence if practice development is to be fully understood. Capturing the essence of this interplay offers nurse researchers a major challenge in the coming years especially as $SI = f(E,C,F)$ is potentially a dynamic system. The actions of the facilitator will influence the context while the context will influence the nature of the evidence that can be assembled to evaluate the effectiveness of practice development. The relationship therefore between these three variables and the successful implementation of change may not follow the linear path as suggested by Kitson et al. (1998). It may actually be a chaotic system indicating that small changes in any of these three characteristics could have major and unpredictable outcomes in practice development terms. The next chapter will explore strategies for change. It will bring together the issues of individual practice development that have featured in early chapters with organizational strategies based upon change theory. In this way I hope to bring the book to a close with some indications at least as to ways forward which might achieve some success in practice development for nursing.

References

Clarke, J. (1999). Evidence Based Practice; a retrograde step? The importance of pluralism in evidence generation for the practice of health care. *Journal of Clinical Nursing*, **8**, 1, 89–94.

Cheater, F. and Closs, J. (1997). The effectiveness of methods of dissemination and implementation of clinical guidelines for nursing practice; a review. *Clinical Effectiveness in Nursing*, **1**, 14–15.

Christian, S. and Norman, I. (1998). Clinical leadership in nursing development units. *Journal of Advanced Nursing*, **27**, 1, 108–116.

French, K. (1981). Methodological considerations in hospital patient opinion surveys. *International Journal of Nursing Studies*, **18**, 7–32.

Funk, S. and Champagne, M. (1991). Barriers; the barriers to research implementation scale. *Applied Nursing Research*, **4**, 2, 90–95.

Greenwood, J. (1999). Clinical Development Units (Nursing); the Western Sydney approach. *Journal of Advanced Nursing*, **28**, 3, 674–679.

Kitson, A., Harvey, G. and McCormack, B. (1998). Enabling the implementation of evidence based practice: a conceptual framework. *Quality in Health Care*, **7**, 149–158.

McColl, E., Bond, S. and Thomas, L. (1996). A study to determine patient satisfaction with nursing care. *Nursing Standard*, **10**, 52, 34–38.

Newman, M., Papadopoulous, I. and Sigsworth, J. (1998). Barriers to evidence based practice. *Clinical Effectiveness in Nursing*, **2**, 1, 11–20.

Nursing Standard (1998). NDU effects on patients not known (news report). **12**, 24, 9.

Ovretveit, J. (1992). *Health Service Quality*. Oxford: Blackwell Science.

Page, S., Allsopp, D. and Casley, S. (1998). *The Practice Development Unit*. London: Whurr Publishers.

Redfearn, S. and Stevens, W. (1998). Nursing Development Units, their structure and orientation. *Journal of Clinical Nursing*, **7**, 218–226.

Thomas, L., McColl, E., Priest, J., Bond, S. and Boys, R. (1996). Newcastle satisfaction with nursing scales; an instrument for quality assessment of nursing care. *Quality in Health Care*, **5**, 67–72.

Thomas, L. (1999). Clinical practice guidelines. *Evidence Based Nursing*, **2**, 2, 38–39.

Tinkler, A., Hotchkiss, J., Nelson, A. and Edwards, L. (1999). Implementing evidence based leg ulcer management. *Evidence Based Nursing*, **2**, 1, 6–8.

Walsh, M. (1997). How nurses perceive barriers to research implementation. *Nursing Standard*, **11**, 29, 34–39.

Ward, M., Titchen, A. and Morrel, C. (1998). Using a supervisory framework to support and evaluate a multiproject practice development programme. *Journal of Clinical Nursing*, **7**, 29–36.

Whitman, W. (1855). Song of Myself. In: Heaney, S. and Hughes, T. (eds) (1997) *The School Bag*. London: Faber and Faber.

Wright, S. and Salvage, J. (1995). *Nursing Development Units; A Force for Change*. London: RCN Publications.

CHAPTER 9

Understanding change

On you go now! Run, son, like the devil
And tell your mother to try
To find me a bubble for the spirit level
And a new knot for this tie

Seamus Heaney, *The Errand*

Introduction

The key to successful change can be as elusive as the errand on which
Seamus Heaney's young boy was dispatched. There is no easy formula
which, if followed, will guarantee success and open the doors to practice
development. However, there are basic principles which guide change
and which at least increase the probabilities of success. This chapter will
explore some of these strategies as developing and advancing nursing
practice must involve change. This will occur initially at the level of the
individual nurse and patient, but changes here will have an effect upon
how the whole team of nurses and the wider multidisciplinary team work
together. This in turn has organizational implications at unit/departmen-
tal/practice level and ultimately on up to Trust/Primary Care Group and
national policy levels. You cannot escape the interconnectedness of real
life and the ensuing complexity that produces. This was a major theme
which we explored in the preceding chapter. Finding solutions to
problems of change at multiple levels is therefore essential for practice
development to occur. While it may appear as elusive as shopping for a
bubble in a spirit level, adherence to the principles outlined below will
make the task less daunting.

Basic models of change

Authors such as Ford and Walsh (1994) and Wright (1998) have reviewed,
summarized and placed in a nursing context some of the basic theory
about change which can be found in management textbooks. There are

three basic models of change and they should be studied in conjunction with the section on the culture of organizations (Chapter 2). As we have seen, organizational culture consists of the values, attitudes and beliefs that are widespread within an organization. Culture therefore is a major determinant of behaviour and, as such, important in understanding change. The three broad approaches to change can be summarized as:

- ❑ The Power–Coercive Model
- ❑ The Rational–Empirical Model
- ❑ The Normative–Educative Model.

The power-coercive model can be summarized by the phrase 'top-down'. In other words the initiative for change comes from senior management who issue new policy statements or instructions and expect junior staff lower down the hierarchy to implement the change. This is a familiar model to all who work in the NHS and fits with either a power or a role culture (Zeus and Apollo respectively, see p. 27). Staff are not involved in the change process other than as passive and obedient servants. Such directives might tell you what you have to do but rarely tell you how to do it; consequently there are major implementation problems and staff do not feel they own the change. Their expertise is not valued in any way and possible solutions to problems are missed because nobody in authority bothered to ask the staff who work with the problems in the real world on a day to day basis. The power-coercive model also has a strong element of arrogance about it and reflects something of the assumptions made by its practitioners about the world around them. Macho managers assume superiority by virtue of occupational group, gender, position in the hierarchy, qualifications held, rank or prestige to name but a few. Expertise in clinical practice, good interpersonal communication and motivational skills are usually conspicuous by their absence. The result is often the *appearance* of change (although nothing much has really changed at any depth) and a disgruntled workforce. If you want a good example of this model in action, reflect upon the way the nursing process was introduced or, more recently, the massive changes made in the NHS as a result of the Conservative Government's market reforms.

The rational-empirical model is based upon the notion that if management explains the changes that have to be made, presenting evidence to support their view, staff can be persuaded to change their practice. This is still largely a top-down approach. It sounds a more user-friendly approach than the power-coercive model and at least affords the nurse the respect of being treated as an intelligent human being who has worthwhile knowledge and skills. The problem with this model is that human beings are not rational and logical all the time and therefore not always prone to persuasion. All sorts of fears and anxieties come into play. Attitudes and belief systems are not changed by rational argument and persuasion. If they were, people would not display racist attitudes or indulge in religious bigotry, they would not smoke, drink excess alcohol, drive too fast, overeat or indulge in irresponsible sex, to name but a few aspects of life. Nurses are as prone to these flaws as anybody else (although hopefully not to the same extent).

The normative-educative model is sometimes called a bottom-up approach as the intent is to produce change by securing the participation of as many staff as possible. It recognizes that the staff themselves have much vital knowledge which is essential for effective change to occur. The staff group is therefore encouraged to propose its own ideas for change and work out its own strategy for implementation. The staff therefore own and are committed to the change. Success acts as positive reinforcement and can lead on to the staff tackling bigger projects. Problems arise, however, if the staff do not have the skills to work out solutions or if they do not appreciate the impact of their ideas beyond their own immediate clinical area. Facilitation is the key to resolving these problems.

Not surprisingly it is this normative-educative, bottom-up approach to change which has won the support of nurse leaders. It offers empowerment for staff and a way of including patients in the change process. The NDU/PDU movements have embraced this as a model for change but as we saw on p. 125 they have found the going tough. Problems of the context within which staff groups have tried to make changes have hindered practice development. This underlines the importance of culture in change. The proposal by Kitson *et al.* (1998) that successful implementation of practice development is a function of evidence, context and facilitation is consistent with both the theory and practice of change reviewed so far (p. 131).

Change and the individual

If we are to make changes in practice which reflect the dramatic advancement and expansion of nursing that potentially could happen, we need a deeper analysis of change than provided in the brief summary given so far. A good place to start is with individuals as these are the building blocks of teams. How individuals might respond to change is an essential insight we must have, to work with the normative-educative model of change.

There are two simple questions to start with when facing the need to change and develop practice. First, ask whether the change comes from within the group or is it imposed from outside? Secondly, ask how much control the group has over the change? It is essential to clarify whose idea the change is at the very beginning as this can avoid a lot of confusion and misunderstanding later.

A key concept in understanding change is the notion that individuals vary enormously in their willingness to change. Oldcorn (1996) summarizes this continuum of change with a helpful diagram (Figure 9.1).

In any group of staff it is possible to find some or all these attitudes towards change. There are no hard and fast boundaries between these categories just as there are no hard boundaries in the colours of the spectrum; they blur into one another. This point about boundaries has

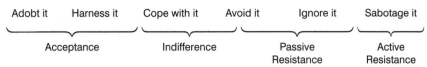

Figure 9.1 How people deal with change

already been made in general terms (p. 110). The nurse who wishes to develop practice whether it be as an individual, or with his or her team, has to recognize that this spectrum of responses exists. He or she also has to ask who is the group affected by the change as it may be wider than he or she at first thinks? People who are at the acceptance end of the spectrum will either adopt the change and ensure its implementation or will see the change as useful to themselves and therefore go along with change, harnessing it for themselves.

It is important to check with people that, in the process of implementation or 'harnessing', other agendas are not being introduced which might confuse the issue. This relates back to the point about where the origin of the change is located. Nurses might want to introduce a nurse practitioner fast track scheme into A&E so that patients with minor conditions can be seen more rapidly. Casualty officers may willingly accept the change but seek to harness it for their own benefit and alter their shift rosters without telling the nursing staff. If such a communication failure occurs there can be unforeseen consequences and misunderstandings within the department. Discussion between medical and nursing staff can, however, allow changes in the medical rosters to occur without any detrimental effect upon the whole department. Another real example involves NHS Direct, which has been introduced to benefit patients. Some GPs may be tempted to harness this change to benefit themselves by diverting out of hours calls to that service. NHS Direct was not intended to be a substitute for GP emergency on-call schemes. Patients may become very irate when told to see their GP by the nurse on the end of the phone having just been told to ring the NHS Direct Nurse by their GP's answering machine. Acceptance of change, however welcome, should not be taken at face value without checking whether people are harnessing change to their own benefit and, in the process, altering or undermining the whole point of the exercise.

A common attitude to change is that, 'It won't affect me', leading to indifference and avoidance strategies such as being too busy to deal with it. This attitude is dangerous when displayed by those in leadership positions such as ward sisters, especially if the change has originated outside the work group or organization. By the time such people have become aware of what is happening it is too late to modify events and the best that can be done is to find ways of coping. Nurses are familiar with this scenario which leads to a position of learned helplessness. We just expect change to happen and we passively react by learning to cope rather than being proactive and steering change from the beginning. Consider the example of setting up new services, moving to a new building or closing down a service. Nurses should not be passively waiting to be told what to do or to be redeployed. They must become involved from the outset and not just fall back on the rationalization that this is all management and nothing to do with them. Such an attitude of course allows nursing to disclaim responsibility for events, all the blame can be shuffled off onto 'management', whoever they are. That is not the practice of the accountable professional that we like to think we are as nurses.

Resisters to change can either be passive or active. At least with someone who is actively resisting change you know who is against the proposals which gives you a chance to work on the problem. When the senior radiographer refuses to allow nurses to authorize X-rays, you at least know who the problem is and by discussion can find out why it is a problem for this person. This then allows you to develop a strategy aimed at changing that person's opinion. We will discuss such strategies later. More difficult, however, are the passive resisters who will not say 'no' but who will not implement change either. It is often very difficult to identify such individuals as they blend into the background, doing nothing to attract attention to themselves. It is important to check out any assumptions that you may have made in developing change as they may go astray due to passive and therefore invisible resistance. Having set up your fast track nurse practitioner service in A&E (or primary health care) you may find it cannot be sustained because so few patients appear to want to use it. The problem might be that the reception staff do not like the idea and simply fail to inform patients that they have the option of seeing a nurse practitioner. They are not actively resisting change but, by doing nothing, they are undermining the change.

Oldcorn (1996) has remarked that what people really resist are the implications of change rather than the change itself. This is a useful insight as in expanding practice you should always be thinking beyond the immediate obvious changes in role and asking yourself what the implications of these changes are. This becomes particularly important when you start to consider other people who will become involved; how will they perceive the implications of change?

One important implication of a nurse expanding her role might be that doctors will feel threatened, perceiving nursing to be trying to take over medicine. They may feel their clinical skills are devalued if a nurse can take on a role that was previously thought to be medical. It is the implications of this that might lead a doctor to say, 'I spent 5 years at medical school getting two degrees to learn to do this and here you are with an RGN qualification saying you can take over my role.' Another example comes from the developing nurse practitioner role in A&E or primary health care. One possible implication of the need for the NP to see as many patients as possible is that he or she will ask other nurses to carry out dressings or give injections for him or her once the patient has been assessed, and the NP has decided what the problem is and what should be done about it. However, some practice nurses or A&E staff nurses may resent the NP acting in this way and tell the NP to do their own dressings! We have to think through the implications of change very carefully if we are to understand resistance to change and avoid the sort of conflict outlined above.

There are several factors that can contribute to making a person resist change and/or being alarmed at the implications that change may bring. Oldcorn (1996) suggests the following:

❏ The person's general attitude to change and their beliefs and values. Attitudes, beliefs and values form stable patterns in people and tend to be closely linked to behaviour. Attitudes, beliefs and values are the essence of culture and there is a strong feedback loop between culture and behaviour. Certain cultures produce certain behaviours which, in turn, reinforce the culture (Ford and Walsh, 1994). As a generalization, if a person is conservative and suspicious of change in one area, they are likely to be like that in most other aspects of life. The converse is also likely to be true.

❏ Feelings of insecurity. The major upheavals that have beset the NHS in the last decade or so have generated such fears in many staff. These are not only structural changes such as Trusts, Fund Holding Practices, Primary Care Groups etc., but also attempts to impose new cultural values from the top, such as the failed experiment with market forces. Nurses have found themselves being served with redundancy notices, their salary and grade arbitrarily reduced as part of cost cutting measures or their workplace simply closed as an 'efficiency' saving. Events such as this, which have been extensively reported by the media and highlighted by politicians when it has suited them, all contributed to a climate of insecurity and declining morale during the 1990s. These are only examples of change from within the NHS to which must be added changes taking place outside the NHS in the very fabric of society. Examples include the changing age distribution in the population which is one very predictable change that still seems to have caught the NHS by surprise, while the increasing health problems caused by drug abuse and social exclusion still remain to be grappled with.

❏ Relationships with the organization and immediate leadership. If a nurse has confidence in his or her organization, feels valued and respected, then he or she will feel more confident and secure, leading to easier acceptance of change. Sadly the experience of the last decade or more has left many nurses battered and bruised, overworked and exhausted. Morale is at an all time low and thousands of nursing posts remain unfilled while universities struggle to attract new recruits. It is against this background, which has seen the NHS gain the reputation of being one of the worst employers in the country, that we have to look at staff–management relationships. There are encouraging signs that with the abolition of the internal market and a fresh approach from the New Labour government elected in 1997, that things may slowly start to improve. At local level, however, things can be turned around more quickly. If you want staff to tackle change constructively there have to be good interpersonal working relationships, trust and open communication. Staff have to feel valued, respected and important, none of which need cost money. If staff hold their leader in high regard, change is more readily accomplished. The NHS badly needs to invest in developing clinical leaders and it remains to be seen whether the newly proposed Nurse Consultant grade is allowed to develop into a cadre of clinical leaders or becomes just another tier of middle management.

❏ Previous experience of change. Unhappy and painful change experiences such as losing your job or having to reapply for your own job against internal competition are not conducive to approaching further change with open arms. The NHS tradition of top-down, power-coercive change leads to learned helplessness in the face of change. Previous experience is again acting as a barrier to a more inclusive bottom-up model.

We can begin to gain insights into the problems faced in introducing innovative nursing roles from consideration of the key individual factors discussed above. However, the real world is about how people interact with each other in the workplace and, as we have said in the previous chapter, the total is more than the sum of the individual parts. Understanding the barriers to change therefore requires more than just looking at individuals in the workplace and simply summing their individual characteristics. We have to look at how they interrelate to each other and the wider organization.

Change and the workplace environment

The culture of the workplace has already been identified as one of the key factors in understanding change. There are, however, two ways of looking at culture; it can be understood in either structural or inter-pretative terms (Wilson, 1992). The structuralist view of culture has already been discussed and is exemplified by the views of Handy (1995). He lists four broad types of organization that are recognizable by their structures as being hierarchical and role-centred; dominated by one powerful individual; consisting of small teams working on their own problems in a matrix structure; or a loose association of individuals with no real structure at all (p. 27). Each of these structures arises out of the workplace and in turn determines the behaviour of the workplace so that organizational cultures tend to be self-propagating entities that are very resistant to change (Williams *et al.*, 1989).

In an interpretative perspective on organizational culture, we are concerned with the symbols used to denote status and membership, the language used and how people act out their roles. The health service is full of symbolism. Consider nursing's obsession with uniform: the traditional nurses' uniform is a Victorian maid's outfit which speaks volumes for nursing's position in the order of things. Yet nurses still long for their uniform, and having got their dress they then want to differentiate themselves from all the other nurses by virtue of colour or some other badge or insignia. Medical staff don their white coats to distinguish themselves from everybody else for there is no other practical reason to wear a white coat. It offers no protection against body fluids, is hot in summer and hardly keeps out the cold in winter. If the white coat is abandoned, medical staff still feel they have to have a badge of office and so the stethoscope is casually slung around the back of the neck just in case people do not realize that they are doctors. A prominent identity badge with a clear photograph would suffice to identify any member of staff and with far more security than a coloured dress or a white coat.

The importance of this issue is striking, as a common theme in the author's experience of nurses developing their roles has always been uniforms. Much time has been spent debating whether the nurse should wear a nurse's dress, plain clothes or a white coat in her new role. So far, the white coat is usually rejected indicating the nurse does not wish to be identified with that most potent of medical symbols. Often plain clothes are chosen almost as a way of the nurse distancing herself from her traditional nursing role. This contrasts with my experiences of visiting the Regional University Hospital (RiTø) at Tromsø in northern Norway where all staff, regardless of grade and position, wear the same uniform (basically a pair of white pyjamas!) distinguishing themselves only by identity badge. The culture of Scandinavian countries is much more egalitarian than the UK and nursing and medical staff in Tromsø are mildly amused at the preoccupation of the British with rank, status and uniform. There is a much more equal feel to the relationships among staff in this particular large teaching hospital than in any equivalent hospital I have worked in, in the UK.

The uniforms we wear are powerful evidence that Wilson (1992) is right to stress the symbolism and interpretation of culture. There are many other examples which the reader might reflect upon including the oft heard phrase dropping quite naturally from medical lips, '*My* nurses will (or will not). . . '. This little phrase can be linked to its other variant, '*My* patients need . . . '. The concept of personal ownership of another human being was abolished with the slave trade yet we still find doctors talking quite normally in these terms. These phrases convey powerful meanings concerning the perceived order of things as seen from a medical viewpoint. A doctor would never say that he *owns* a nurse or a patient, it is not as simplistic as that. However, there is this assumption that medicine is in overall control of all things; how else can the word 'my' be interpreted? This medical perception of 'my' patient has to be recognized in working with medicine to expand nursing roles.

One final example of how symbols and signs speak volumes about the culture of the NHS may be found in the hospital car park. Logically it is those staff who have to drive in to work at unsociable hours when it is often dark who should be able to park their cars closest to the hospital entrance in well lit secure areas, particularly if they are female. In other words nursing staff and other on-call technical staff such as radiographers and laboratory technicians. Have a look at your hospital main entrance next time you go to work, those prime car parking spaces usually have prominent signs on them reserving them for senior managers and consultants, the very people who least need secure well lit convenient car parking. Nursing staff and others are probably banished to the furthest corners of the car park! This speaks volumes about where the power lies and the perceptions of those who hold it.

In planning changes and development of the nursing role it is important therefore to be on the look out for such clues about culture. It is not only the structures of an organization that matter but also the interpretative perspective. The symbols and meanings that are attached to them and the systems that are used to get things done tell us a great deal about an organization's culture, whether it be at unit or Trust level. (See Chapter 2 for a discussion of the McKinsey 7S analysis which is very relevant to this discussion.) The interpretative standpoint is particularly important as in the previous section we emphasized that resistance to change is more likely to be due to the individual's perceptions of the implications of change rather than the actual change itself. How the individual sees things therefore is the key and to understand this we have to look at how the individual fits into the culture just as much as looking at the interplay between culture and organizational structure.

Purely structural solutions to problems of change will not work. As Wilson (1992) explains, simply dismantling a bureaucratic structure will not lead to change unless you also address issues of ideology, inter-personal relationships, roles and symbols. The McKinsey 7S analysis that we discussed earlier in this book (Chapter 2) makes exactly the same point; changing structures alone will not lead to change unless you change the other six Ss such as systems, staff, skills etc. New nursing roles cannot be introduced without addressing the complex cultural issues of symbolism, systems of working, and how individuals interpret the organization in which they work.

The interaction of the individual and the workplace

It is now time to bring these two topics together and look what happens when they meet. According to McCalman and Paton (1992) change problems can be classified as either hard or soft. Their analysis is congruent with the differentiation into structural and interpretative views of culture. A hard change problem is therefore about systems and structures, whereas a soft problem is a more subjective, organizational development issue. Perhaps better terms than hard and soft would be clear cut and fuzzy respectively. Table 9.1 shows the differences.

'Hard' change problems are more likely to occur in the Trust finance office or stores department when new methods of accounting or ordering are introduced. The 'soft' problems are, however, the sort faced by clinicians and, paradoxically, it could be argued are much harder (i.e. more difficult) than the 'hard' problems! Solutions for these 'soft' problems require a great deal of interpersonal skill from all involved

Table 9.1 'Hard' and 'soft' problems

Hard	Soft
Quantifiable objectives, clear performance objectives and indicators	Subjective, at best semi-quantifiable performance indicators
Systems/technical orientation	People orientation
Small number of possible solutions	Wide range of possible solutions
Clearly defined problem	Unclear definition of problem
Resource requirements clear	Resource requirements not clear
Static environment	Changing environment
Known time scales	Fuzzy or open ended time scale
Clear boundaries to problem with minimal external interactions	Indistinct boundaries with many possible external factors at work

Adapted from McCalman and Paton (1992)

especially the leaders, as possible solutions will generate conflicts of interest. There is no cookbook recipe approach to solving such change problems. The warning against drawing neat boundaries between categories is still in operation here, however. In reality hard and soft problems are not two totally distinct groups, they have a grey area where they merge into each other.

On p. 143 we stressed that being clear where the origins of change lie was crucial to a successful outcome. It is worth now returning to that point as it has a major impact upon how the individual views change (and the organization too for that matter). The source of change and the individual's likely attitudes are summarized in Table 9.2.

Table 9.2 Relationship between attitudes to change and the source of change

Internally generated change	Externally generated change
Proactive stance	Reactive responses
Positive feelings	Negative feelings
Greater driving forces for change	Greater restraining forces holding change back
Viewed as an opportunity that could be exploited	Viewed as a problem to be solved
Greater control and therefore certainty	Greater uncertainty and therefore less control
Less disruption to practice	More disruption
Closed boundaries and fixed time scales	Indistinct boundaries and fuzzy time scales

Adapted from McCalman and Paton (1992)

The list of attitudes in the right hand column are familiar to many nurses as this is often how change appears to them. The reason is obvious; nurses usually have change imposed upon them from outside the nursing team. The left hand column appears to be a much more positive way of looking at change and can be arrived at providing change is coming from within nursing utilizing the normative-educative model summarized on p. 142. The implications of McCalman and Paton's analysis is that if change can be addressed as an internal issue, i.e. change coming from within the clinical team, then it is more likely to succeed even if it is usually of the complex 'soft' variety shown in Table 9.1. Ownership is therefore the key to determining how favourable an individual's attitude is likely to be to change. A key factor for success in change is to get all the staff involved and to ensure they have a shared perception of the issues at stake. If ownership is combined with the knowledge that the staff also control the immediate surrounding environment within which the change is located, this creates very favourable conditions for change. If those higher placed in a hierarchical structure (such as the NHS) control the change environment this mitigates against change, particularly if they are driving the change in a top-down manner.

Managers who would wish to encourage practice development should therefore encourage staff to develop their own ideas for change and also delegate authority to staff to manage their own affairs if the conditions for success described above are to be achieved. A balance has to be struck by managers between a hands off approach and being supportive when needed. The clinical governance agenda stresses the importance of bringing decision making closer to the patient. If this aspiration can be translated into practice it will create a more change friendly environment by virtue of empowering staff to initiate change themselves in an environment they control. This discussion emphasizes again the importance of the context to the successful implementation of practice development (p. 134).

Although wherever possible change should come from within a staff group and nurses should be proactive in steering change, it sometimes does happen that change comes from an external source. The importance of outside stimuli is argued by Wilson (1992). He considers that the institutionalized fabric of organizations acts to resist change until one of the following scenarios occurs:

❏ The advent of new data or technology to which the organization is unaccustomed. In the nursing context new technology could be a new dressing, a surgeon performing a new operation or a new medicine.
❏ Increasing conflict between powerful stakeholders. The emerging Primary Care Groups will be powerful stakeholders in how hospital services are delivered and their views may be at odds with the conventional approach of hospital staff. There is a real danger that hospital nurses in particular are already adopting an attitude of indifference leading to avoidance of this issue (see Figure 9. 1) which could have serious consequences in the near future.

❏ A novel topic presents itself with which the organization has not had to deal before but which demands a decision. Closing down services is one such example that has happened in the recent past.

❏ There is an unusual or unexpected source of new ideas which breaks through traditional lines of communication to open up new discussions. Many ideas to expand nursing roles might be thought of in these terms, particularly with reference to the nurse practitioner concept which repeatedly brings nurses and doctors together in new ways. It might even be suggested that the consultant nurse idea comes into this category as it appeared to have originated in No.10 Downing Street and bypassed the Department of Health on its way to a public announcement at the 1998 Nurse of the Year Awards!

❏ The onset of crisis. This category has been typical of the NHS for far too long. It is to be hoped that the Labour Government will replace the short-term outlook, that was so characteristic of the Conservative Government's policy towards the NHS, with a stable and adequately funded operational environment.

As nurses develop and expand their roles, we need to realize that while ideally we should be doing so proactively from within nursing, external factors such as these can make such an impact upon the care environment that they do produce change. A key notion in Wilson's analysis is resistance to change and forces that can impact upon the organization to produce change. This conjures up a picture of a school laboratory science experiment aimed at understanding the basic laws of dynamics and forces. Something like this picture must have presented itself to Kurt Lewin who, nearly 50 years ago, described a very simple model to allow the conceptualization of change in just such terms (Lewin, 1951). His force field model of change has stood the test of time and is still used today as a simple but effective way of understanding the powers at play in any change problem.

Lewin postulates that the status quo can be represented by a straight line. There are two sets of forces at work in maintaining the status quo, drivers for change and resisters to change. To understand the mechanics of the situation he suggests that you list the forces on either side of the status quo line, representing each one by a line whose length is directly proportional to its strength (Figure 9.2). The change process now consists of unfreezing this status quo to allow movement to occur and then refreezing the changed situation. Refreezing is essential if the change is not to unravel and people slide back to their old ways. Unfreezing the situation therefore takes place by either increasing the forces driving for change and/or weakening the forces resisting change to such an extent that the status quo can no longer hold and the balance of forces is destabilized.

Oldcorn (1996) and McCalman and Paton (1992) offer the following helpful suggestions for ways to undermine resistance to change:

❏ Show that change has the full support of senior management.

❏ The ideas come from the people who have to make the changes. This reiterates the theme of group ownership and a

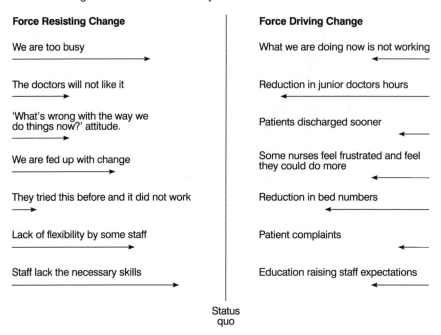

Force Resisting Change	Force Driving Change
We are too busy	What we are doing now is not working
The doctors will not like it	Reduction in junior doctors hours
'What's wrong with the way we do things now?' attitude.	Patients discharged sooner
We are fed up with change	Some nurses feel frustrated and feel they could do more
They tried this before and it did not work	Reduction in bed numbers
Lack of flexibility by some staff	Patient complaints
Staff lack the necessary skills	Education raising staff expectations

Status
quo

Figure 9.2 Lewin's force field theory of change. An illustrative example based on many typical examples

shared vision of the change process. It also makes the change appear to be internally driven which will produce less opposition than externally imposed change.

❑ There is something in it to benefit those involved, e.g. it appears to reduce workload.

❑ If it does not threaten job security or salary.

❑ Make the idea sound interesting or exciting.

❑ If the change is in harmony with the values and beliefs of the staff.

❑ Economic incentives on their own are rarely enough to bring about change unless the main resistance is only on economic grounds.

❑ There is good communication and flow of information to all involved.

The discussion on practice development (Chapter 4) should be read with these thoughts in mind. The work undertaken by Steve Wright and myself on practice development by networking has stuck close to these principles and so have successful NDU/PDU projects. The first two points in this list cannot be emphasized enough however. The following ideas may be put on the other side of the force field diagram as factors that will increase the drive for change:

❑ Specific information relevant to daily practice will have more impact than generalizations about national statistics, e.g. readmission rates or waiting lists.

❏ A group with continuing psychological meaning will have more influence than an *ad hoc* temporary collection of individuals. In other words try to work with existing teams of staff who know each other and who will continue to work with each other after the change occurs.

❏ Identify individuals within groups who are seen as leaders and who enjoy high prestige. They are the most influential and winning them over early can pay big dividends in persuading others to adopt the changes proposed. Such people may not be the official leaders such as managers with the most seniority. They may be charismatic individuals who are quite junior in the hierarchy or very experienced staff who have worked in the area for many years.

❏ Keep people well informed at all times.

❏ Get the group fully involved so that they come to own the change.

❏ Offer the change as a reversible option. If staff do not like it or it does not work, we can go back to the old ways or try something else. This approach therefore requires a strong research element to the project to evaluate how it is proceeding against agreed criteria for success.

❏ An incremental approach is more acceptable but you should beware the risk of missing opportunities by being too cautious.

❏ Investigate whether individuals are ready and willing to tackle change. Give them the training they need to be involved in change and also to develop their own practice.

❏ Deal sensitively with individuals at all times especially if their position in the new order of things is doubtful.

Figure 9.3 shows how these factors may be translated into real examples such as introducing a multidisciplinary patient held record on a younger disabled unit (YDU), while Figure 9.4 shows the same approach applied to the problem of introducing a nurse practitioner run orthopaedic preoperative assessment clinic. Both examples relate to changes made at the West Cumberland Hospital, Whitehaven.

In order to unfreeze the situation educational staff from St Martins College (Lawrence Harper, Anna Walsh) and Steve Wright worked with the YDU staff over a period of several months. The following techniques were used which can be related to the sort of strategies outlined by Oldcorn above. Regular meetings and good communication ensured a high level of staff ownership and participation. This allowed exploration of the medicolegal issues with staff and networking with other parts of the country allowed us to introduce the unit to staff who had made the change to patient held records. This allayed many fears about what might happen which were understandably acting as change resisters. A multidisciplinary document was drawn up with facilitation by St Martins staff and introduced, but only on the basis that it would be piloted first (reversible change) and evaluated using the research skills of St Martins staff. The chief nurse for the Trust lent his support to the project and it quickly became apparent in the group development work that this would

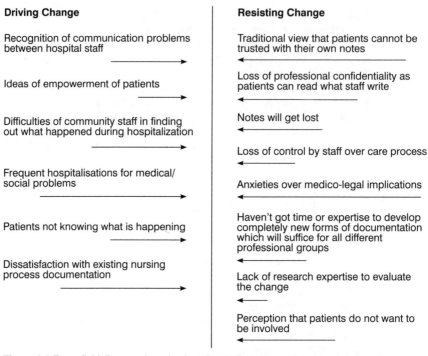

Driving Change

Recognition of communication problems between hospital staff
──────────────▶

Ideas of empowerment of patients
──────────▶

Difficulties of community staff in finding out what happened during hospitalization
──────────────▶

Frequent hospitalisations for medical/ social problems
──────────────▶

Patients not knowing what is happening
──────────▶

Dissatisfaction with existing nursing process documentation
──────────────▶

Resisting Change

Traditional view that patients cannot be trusted with their own notes
◀──────────────

Loss of professional confidentiality as patients can read what staff write
◀──────────

Notes will get lost
◀──────

Loss of control by staff over care process
◀────

Anxieties over medico-legal implications
◀──────────────

Haven't got time or expertise to develop completely new forms of documentation which will suffice for all different professional groups
◀────

Lack of research expertise to evaluate the change
◀────

Perception that patients do not want to be involved
◀──────────

Figure 9.3 Force field diagram: introduction of multidisciplinary patient held documentation (YDU)

have major advantages for all concerned. A strong multidisciplinary culture existed already on the unit which was very helpful as this meant the proposed changes were in line with the beliefs and values of the staff.

The document was introduced and evaluated by means of telephone follow-up interviews with carers which showed it was well received. Minor modifications were made and the document is now in its second year of use by the YDU. A significant and successful change in practice had been accomplished by means of strengthening forces driving change and weakening those that resisted change. Outside facilitation had played a key part in this change, operating within a positive culture and drawing upon evidence from elsewhere showing this was a possible and successful change to make to practice. The three elements of the Kitson *et al.* (1998) model were all in place, combined with a force field analysis. The result was successful change.

A key point concerning culture in this example was that a multi-disciplinary culture already existed. If you are considering setting up a PDU, this multidisciplinary culture has to be there to improve your chances of success. A valuable tool in this connection is the Team Climate Inventory (TCI) of Anderson and West (1994) which has been developed in a range of public service settings. This tool gives a reliable indication of the extent to which team work is developed within a group of staff and was used by Walsh and Walsh (1998) in researching an attempt to set up a PDU on a general surgical ward. The TCI demonstrated a series of low scores on the various measures of teamwork indicating the staff were not really functioning as a truly multidisciplinary team. They were working in a fairly traditional way in which they got along with each other in a polite, civil way but did not really engage each other's practice with a shared vision and goal. The attempt at obtaining PDU accreditation failed and was abandoned shortly after the TCI research was carried out. Walsh and Walsh concluded that the TCI was a valuable diagnostic tool for assessing the strength of teamwork in a unit. This is a crucial element in deciding whether to go for PDU status or defer such a move until some serious team building activity has taken place.

In the example shown in Figure 9.4, the status quo of conventional GP referral to orthopaedic outpatients, medical assessment, placing on the waiting list and subsequent admission for surgery was placed under increasing pressure by external events. These are familiar nationally and summarized by the first three items under drivers for change. However, the resisters were so strong, particularly the medical tradition, that for a while nothing happened. The situation was unfrozen when the availability of a BSc Nurse Practitioner programme locally, which was championed by the nursing management of the hospital, was added to the growing pressures for change. A lot of joint planning and group work took place to develop the NP-run preoperative assessment clinic. An incremental approach to change was adopted allowing the NP gradually to increase her scope of practice and authority, linked to her progression on the course. One of the hospital consultants acted as her medical facilitator (a clinical tutor role which is required as part of the BSc Nurse Practitioner course), which had the beneficial effect of involving the medical staff fully in her clinical skills development. The clinical audit department has been carefully monitoring her work to evaluate its effectiveness. The team developing the role were able to persuade medical staff of the potential benefits they would see and experience has confirmed this to be the case.

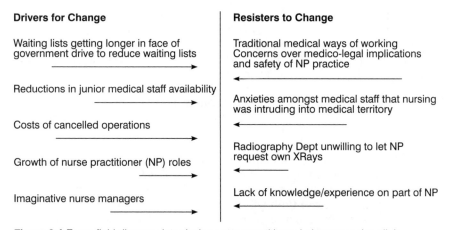

Figure 9.4 Force field diagram: introducing nurse practitioner-led preoperative clinic

A combination of bottom-up change involving all parties from the beginning, an incremental approach underpinned by a high quality educational programme and clinical audit of outcomes has characterized this very successful and innovative development. The force field diagram helps make clear what actually happened. Nursing management played a major role in creating a culture where such changes could occur and the evidence that it was a possible change was also there. External facilitation was less obvious in this example although the involvement of the NP with the BSc programme probably assisted. A great deal of the credit lies with the internal facilitation offered by the NP's immediate manager. The NP-run clinic means that patients are thoroughly assessed before admission. This has dramatically reduced the incidence of patients being admitted who were then found to be unfit for surgery leading to expensive cancellations and delays. It also means that discharge planning can begin before admission takes place, which also increases the efficiency of the service and avoids discharge delays.

Consideration of these examples demonstrates that the force field analysis is a valuable tool in allowing you to visualize the various players and stakeholders involved in making changes to practice. Oldcorn's work (p. 151) also suggests strategies that can be used to unfreeze the situation and make change possible, although this is not an exhaustive list. Local circumstances will lead to various other approaches being used in addition to those listed p. 151. These examples also show the importance of evidence, context and facilitation in the successful (or otherwise) implementation of practice development.

The role of facilitation in developing practice

In the three examples cited above there was strong external facilitation in the case of the YDU, strong internal facilitation in the NP example and no facilitation in the case of the unsuccessful PDU. There is considerable debate about the relative merits of internal and external facilitation and we will return to this point later.

McCalman and Paton (1992) consider that a facilitator needs three key qualities, whether they be an insider or an outsider:

❏ Personality. This involves empathy, listening and interpersonal skills (Kitson *et al.*, (1998) emphasize the importance of these skills)
❏ Analytical and diagnostic skills to identify and work towards problem solutions in the change process. The goal is to help others work out their own solutions rather than do it for them. This is essential if ownership of the development is to occur as it has to come from within rather be imposed from outside
❏ Client related experience. This is essential in order to have the understanding of the problem needed to apply the skills listed

under the two previous points. It also gives the facilitator credibility in the eyes of the staff with whom he or she is working.

The facilitator therefore has to work in a collaborative style in order to achieve change, as the staff must arrive at their own solutions if the change is to be successfully owned. Solutions also need to be put into practice so the facilitator's role continues through the implementation and evaluation stages.

Facilitation initially involves gathering information about the clinical area and the ideas that are being floated for practice development. These need to be focused into a clear statement summarizing the changes that staff agree are to be made. This ensures that staff are all 'singing from the same hymn sheet' and have a shared view of the change process. The facilitator can make suggestions towards the planned changes, make constructive criticisms, introduce sources of evidence, and put staff in touch with others who have already undertaken similar practice development work. All of this introduces a new perspective on development work as staff may sometimes be too close to the problem to see things differently. Summarizing and integrating different points of view is a vital function for the facilitator during the development process. This involves retaining an overview of the whole project and necessarily a slightly detached point of view in order to ensure objectivity. In multidisciplinary work this is even more important if the views of one professional group are not to become dominant at the expense of others. Continuity is essential during the change process and the facilitator provides this by practical steps such as arranging meetings and circulating notes of previous meetings. He or she also acts as a constant in the equation of change as given the time span of development projects staff inevitably leave and are replaced by others new to the project. Finally, the facilitator has a key role in the evaluation of completed change as feeding this back to all those involved has an important lesson to teach, i.e. how the staff themselves changed practice. This insight will encourage and assist further practice development in the future.

As an outsider, the facilitator has the obvious advantage of objectivity and being outside the power structures of the clinical area. This means you are unaffected by internal politics and much more likely to be *seen as* fair minded and even handed which is just as important as actually *being* fair minded and even handed. Academic staff from the local university nursing faculty have the desirable characteristics of an objective outsider, but they must also have credibility in the eyes of the staff involved. This is another powerful argument for academic staff to engage in clinical practice meaningfully and have an agreed percentage of their time spent in clinical work.

Appointing an internal member of staff to act as facilitator means that person will have to struggle with the problem of being seen as part of the management hierarchy by junior staff. He or she will be close to the problem, possibly too close to see things objectively and may even be part of the problem that requires change to occur. On the other hand, he or she will probably have access to information and background knowledge that an external person will not. McCalman and Paton (1992) consider that there is a golden rule of facilitation which is that, if a person from within the organization is to act in this role, they should never do so in their own area of work. A ward sister or practice nurse therefore should never be expected to facilitate development of practice in their own ward or health centre. This important golden rule underlines the importance of appointing a practice development officer whose job it is to act as a full-time facilitator within the trust or Primary Care Group as these new health care agencies develop.

The literature therefore makes it clear that a facilitator is highly desirable if effective practice development is to occur. Whether the person is internal (employed by the trust or PCG) or external (e.g. an academic from the local university), the relationship between facilitator and facilitated must be a voluntary one based on mutual trust and respect. This means that the facilitation relationship can be severed at any time by either party if things are not working out. The trust or PCG has to recognize that the facilitator is working to improve practice, which implies that there is a problem or at least room for improvement. An open and honest approach is needed rather than being defensive or suspicious of what the person is doing. The relationship is a temporary one, which means that when the project is complete the facilitator will withdraw and move on to another project. The implication is that staff must not become dependent upon the facilitator, one day they will have to stand on their own two feet. If the facilitator has specific skills which are essential to making the changes work, these skills must be passed on to the staff of the unit before he or she leaves. This underlines the importance of education as you cannot develop practice without first developing staff.

The facilitator has to adopt a position akin to that taken by a researcher working in the field of ethnography, i.e. one of marginality. This can be an uncomfortable place to be, but, it is essential to get the balance right between being close enough to understand what is happening and not being too close so as to lose objectivity ('going native' as ethnographic researchers sometimes say). There is another balance that has to be struck between being a resource for the change process, i.e. a technical expert with know how and answers to specific questions and being a catalyst for the change process, i.e. a person who helps others to solve their own problems.

Change at strategic level

This chapter has so far concentrated on change at clinical level and found strong evidence to support the model proposed by Kitson *et al.* emphasizing the importance of evidence, context and facilitation in mediating successful change. We will conclude the chapter by looking at the wider picture of strategic change within which local change takes place. As we have already argued these different levels of change are not separate entities but are all interlinked in the natural complexity of the real world.

It is interesting therefore to review the research of Pettigrew *et al.* (1992) who have carried out several studies of strategic change within the NHS. They note that strategic change has proceeded at different rates within the NHS and ask the obvious question, why this should be? Their answer is that it all depends upon the context as they identify receptive and non-receptive contexts within which change can occur. These authors are very critical of much research into change within the NHS for its failure to recognize the importance of context. They argue that change occurs at different levels within an organization and at different times but that it is all interconnected; precisely the point that I argued in the previous chapter. Change does not have a single cause nor does effect follow cause in a simple fashion. Rather there is an interwoven series of feedback loops which means that, in an organization as complicated as the health service, several factors usually combine to cause a change but that change then has several knock on effects which affect the progress of the original change in different ways. Without realizing it Pettigrew *et al.* are describing change in the NHS in terms of complexity theory and are suggesting the ensuing health care is an emergent phenomenon (p. 112).

There is a great deal of support in their findings for the cultural analysis of change we have already presented. They suggest that the key to understanding different rates of change in the NHS lies in differential receptivity, i.e. some areas are more willing to accept and embrace change than others. Change receptive environments have integrative structures and cultures. They are characterized by inter-connectedness, team orientation and cooperative environments which welcome innovation. Good communication, mutual respect and team-work are the key to such cultures. These are contrasted with segmented structures and cultures which are compartmentalized, rule bound hierarchical organizations which smother innovation in a blanket of bureaucracy. The structure and culture of a trust are therefore major determinants of how receptive it is to change. Other factors identified in this research included:

❏ Communication and the sharing of information
❏ Networking
❏ Stability of key personnel who champion change.

There are striking similarities in this work with the account that has been developed so far of the principles that contribute to successful practice development. Pettigrew *et al.* summarize their findings in Figure 9.5. (Pettigrew *et al.*, 1992, p. 276). They deliberately have drawn the diagram with this configuration to make the point that there is no simple cause and effect relationship between any one of these factors and change. They all interrelate with each other and the end product of that complex interaction is the context within which change may occur.

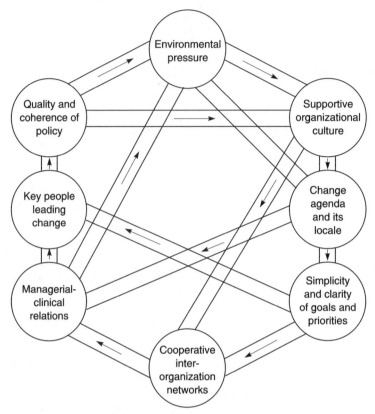

Figure 9.5 Receptive contexts for change: the eight factors

The evidence base for change and the facilitation necessary to act as a catalyst all need superimposition upon this complex contextual diagram.

Summary

This chapter has mapped out the various theoretical perspectives that there are on change and found that there is a convergence of opinion around some key points. Change should ideally be bottom-up using the educative-normative principle. Maximum staff involvement from the very beginning aimed at producing staff ownership and the perception that change is an internal process under the control of staff maximizes the chances of success. Individuals react differently to change and often it is their perceptions of the implications of change that lead to opposition, rather than the change itself. The Lewin force field model has been shown to be a useful tool in understanding change and some useful principles explored that can be applied to different change problems using force field analysis. The importance of context and facilitation are recurring themes running through the literature and practice development is unlikely to succeed without recognition of the role of these two variables, together with evidence. Finally the multifaceted and complex nature of change is reinforced by hard research evidence into strategic change within the NHS.

References

Anderson, N. and West, M. (1994). Team Climate Inventory Questionnaire. Windsor, Berks: NFER-NELSON.

Ford, P. and Walsh, M. (1994). *New Rituals for Old*. Oxford: Butterworth-Heinemann.

Handy, C. (1995). *The Gods of Management*. London: Arrow.

Heaney, S. (1998). *Opened Ground*. London: Faber and Faber.

Kitson, A., Harvey, G. and McCormack, B. (1998). Enabling the implementation of evidence based practice: a conceptual framework. *Quality in Health Care*, **7**, 149–158.

Lewin, K. (1951). *Field Theory in the Social Sciences*. New York: Harper.

McCalman, J. and Paton, R. (1992). *Change Management; A Guide to Effective Implementation*. London: Paul Chapman Publishing.

Oldcorn, R. (1996). *Change Management; A Guide to Effective Implementation*, 3rd edn. London: Macmillan.

Pettigrew, A., Ferlie, E. and McKee, L. (1992). *Shaping Strategic Change*. London: Sage Publications.

Walsh, M. and Walsh, A. (1998). Practice Development Units: a study of teamwork. *Nursing Standard*, **12**, 33, 35–38.

Williams, A., Dobson, P. and Walters, M. (1989). *Changing Culture*. London: Institute of Personnel Managers.

Wilson, D. (1992). *A Strategy of Change*. London: Routledge.

Wright, S. (1998). *Changing Nursing Practice* 2nd edn. London: Arnold.

Moving on

When you are old and grey and full of sleep,
And nodding by the fire, take down this book,
And slowly read, and dream of the soft look
Your eyes had once, and of their shadows deep.

W.B. Yeats (1893) *When you are Old*

Maybe in years to come you will do just as Yeats suggested with this book. I hope you will and, in doing so, look back on a personal career which has seen great changes and developments in nursing. Perhaps you will be able to reflect on changes that you were involved in personally and maybe, just maybe, you will feel this book helped you a little to develop nursing practice. With that optimistic and perhaps mellow thought in mind it is time to recap.

This book began by examining the basic concept of caring which is taken as fundamental to nursing. It then moved on to examine the environment within which those seeking to develop nursing practice have to operate, exploring issues such as accountability, the meaning of professionalism and the legal framework which encompasses nursing. The final chapters have looked at issues related to developing new roles such as the nurse practitioner concept and change theory. It now remains to try to pull this together into a summary which the nurse will find useful in moving practice forward into the future.

Keep focused on the patient

The patient has to remain as the central focus of what we do and why we are here. The UKCC make that point clearly in their various documents. A key test therefore for any new idea is always, how does this benefit the patient? By the same token, whenever practice is under review, a variation on that question should be; is what we are doing now giving the patient the best deal and if not, how can we improve things? The starting point for advancing nursing should always be the patient.

Recognizing where you are coming from and the value of education

The next simple step may sound obvious but is essential to keep development grounded in safe practice. The nurse should always remember that he or she is a nurse. My grandfather was a Dubliner who could have walked out of the pages of a James Joyce novel. He was fond of saying, 'If you want to know the way there, I wouldn't be starting from here.' In other words, where you are starting from in life has a major influence on where you are going.

This has major importance in deciding the direction and extent of practice development as it reminds you that you have a certain level of knowledge behind you together with certain values and assumptions that are unique to nursing. If a new role is overlapping into territory that has traditionally been thought of as the province of medicine, the significance of this observation is that you will have less background in the biological sciences, such as anatomy, physiology and pharmacology, and a different approach to relating to patients from a doctor. The former is a weakness, the latter a strength. The logical approach is therefore to play to your strengths. Cultivate and exploit the advantages that can be gained from maintaining good consultation and communication skills with patients. Allow sufficient time for consultations (not the 5 minute snapshot that is most GP consultations) and give yourself the scope to explore holistically with the patient their health problems rather than zoom in on their ache or pain to the exclusion of everything else.

However much you protect the strengths of the nursing approach, you cannot ignore your weaknesses. This means that education is the key to underpinning practice development as you cannot develop practice without developing yourself. Think of this another way, you do not know what you do not know. Most nurses have real deficits in the areas of the biological sciences compared to doctors. This is hardly surprising as medical schools require good A level results in subjects such as chemistry and biology just to get started. Medical students then study a wide range of biological sciences up to degree standard over a 5-year period. The experienced nurse who has developed his or her practice within a specialized field will certainly have moved his or her own knowledge base a long way forward from their original qualification, however, they will still be lacking in large areas of knowledge when compared to the average doctor.

There is, however, one red herring which needs to be addressed which is the notion that to advance nursing practice you must have a Masters degree. Most medical staff have an education which is at first degree level. There is therefore no logic in expecting nurses to have a qualification at Masters level. I strongly believe that as many nurses as possible should have a degree level education. But if a nurse already has a degree and wishes to undertake a course to expand her area of knowledge then undertaking a second bachelors degree is a perfectly reasonable course of action. This is after all how doctors have trained, taking two bachelors degrees together. There has to be a good reason for undertaking education at Master's level and already having a bachelor's degree is not a good reason! If you want to develop research skills and explore an area of practice from a research perspective, then an MPhil is a good idea. There will be certain specialized areas where a taught Masters will be useful for practice or management, however, in most cases, honours degree level is all that is needed for nursing practice. It would be a sign of professional maturity if nursing recognized this fact. There is no place for 'academic one upmanship' in relation to medicine, which may be behind the desire of some leaders of the nursing profession to place advanced nursing courses at Masters level.

Autonomy is an ideal talked of a great deal by nurses today and in this book I have argued that it is a relative concept only as even the most senior medical consultant no longer enjoys full autonomy. However, developing practice does require increased degrees of autonomy. One of the consequences of which is that the nurse has to stand by his or her decisions without being able to ask for medical back up on every patient seen. Those decisions need to be right, which implies the nurse has to have the knowledge and skills to operate in this increasingly autonomous style. Traditional nurse education has never been geared to produce a practitioner working in such a highly autonomous way, hence the gaps that help to differentiate nursing from medicine. Personal experience working on the BSc Nurse Practitioner course reinforces this view as we have had a fair number of nurses coming on the course confident that they already knew most of what they needed to know to do their jobs, they just wanted it confirmed and to be given the credibility of an honours degree. Every single one of them had changed their mind within 3 months as they began to know what they did not know and realize that there were significant knowledge and skills deficits to be made up.

Nurses developing practice have to recognize the gaps that exist in their knowledge base and rectify them through rigorous and effective education. This will often mean rather more than a few study days organized by the trust training department. A properly accredited course run by an institution of higher education is a more reliable approach to giving the nurse the confidence to practise safely and will enhance the employer's risk management strategy. Medical involvement with such courses is to be welcomed if medicine possesses the relevant knowledge and skills that need to be passed on. Such involvement also has the beneficial effect of improving teamwork and reassuring medical colleagues about the standards reached by the nurse. However, the overall control of the course should remain in nursing hands to be consistent with the philosophy of always remembering that you are a nurse.

It is worth remembering that the law would expect a nurse undertaking a task, which in the past was thought to lie within the medical field of practice, to be as competent as a competent medical practitioner. The patient certainly would have that expectation. Second best is not an option. Managers need to take such points on board and ensure that nurses have appropriate access to education to allow practice development to take place safely. They need to consider the costs to the trust of one single lawsuit for negligence and balance that against the costs of providing effective safe education for nursing staff who are developing their roles.

The development of new roles therefore has to start with identifying the outcomes desired from the role and therefore the skills and knowledge base required for a nurse to practise safely and effectively. This allows the educational requirements of the post holder to be identified and met. It does not, however, require dreaming up a complicated title which seeks to write the nurse's job description on her name badge, nor does it require automatically adopting the much abused 'nurse practitioner' title. Unfortunately, practice development often ends up getting side tracked with trivia such as titles and uniforms which are of secondary importance. What the job entails and how the nurse can be prepared to do it safely are of far greater importance.

Evaluation of practice development

Another issue, which is far more important than titles and uniforms, concerns evaluation of the new role. Establishing a new service or expanding a nurse's role must be accompanied by evaluation to determine the effectiveness of the role. This is more than clinical audit, although clinical audit can play an important part in evaluation. Looking at the new role is a research exercise which should focus on the process of change as well as the outcome (clinical audit is outcome focused and therefore only captures part of the picture). Involving an outside university department in evaluation gives a strong measure of credibility to the results as they will be objective and have no 'axe to grind'. Feedback during the process of change is an accepted part of the action research methodology and captures much valuable information about the process of change which allows fine tuning and alterations to be made. This is unfamiliar territory for many doctors and district ethics committees who are used to the randomized controlled trial (RCT) approach. Tactful explanations of the difference and rationales for adopting such an alternative approach will be useful. Perhaps one way of explaining this different approach to devotees of the RCT is to sell action research methodology as extensive piloting of the interventions before making the final evaluation which could then follow a classic RCT.

It is essential that the NHS builds up a cadre of practitioners who can also carry out research. Involving university departments in researching the effectiveness of new roles therefore should be done in such a way that practitioners learn research skills as part of the exercise. This is far more useful than adopting a 'hired gun' approach which sees an academic mercenary parachute into your unit, do a quick evaluation study and then disappear following the sounds of battle to the next project. Learning partnerships with academia that develop research skills internally for the NHS are the way forward. These may be tied to staff undertaking degrees who can carry out research into the effectiveness of new roles under supervision for their dissertation at first degree or Masters level. They may also research the new role for an MPhil. Such approaches lend themselves to an action research route as the researcher is an integral part of the research setting rather than the outsider normally seen in the RCT. This is why a partnership with academia is needed, as apart from bringing research skills to the scene, the academic also brings the objectivity which only distance can lend.

Working up the idea: professional and legal issues

Implementing a change in practice has to be preceded by a lot of hard work involving refining the idea and gaining the cooperation of all the staff involved. Once the basic outline of the new role has been developed it has to be tested against existing trust/employer policies and UKCC documents such as the *Scope of Professional Practice*. If it clearly goes beyond existing policy then that policy has to be amended to ensure that the nurse is still covered by the principle of vicarious liability whether the employer is a trust, GP or private firm. By the same token, any development should be looked at in conjunction with UKCC requirements starting with the fundamental *Code of Professional Conduct* and also the *Scope of Professional Practice*. The nurse is always accountable to the UKCC. The employer should therefore avoid a clash of interests in this crucial area by only requiring the nurse to operate within UKCC guidelines and codes of practice.

The later chapters in this book introduced some ideas from outside the field of nursing and the social sciences which I believe are very relevant to the creative development of new nursing ideas. In working up the proposal we must not become trapped by boundaries. In the real world, boundaries are an illusion and an artefact that dissolve upon closer inspection just as the colours of the rainbow blur into each other. Green is green and blue is blue, the differences are obvious but, as they merge into each other, the boundary between these colours is not. So it is with practice, medicine is medicine and nursing is nursing, but at the boundary they merge into each other. We need to recognize that in developing new nursing roles such as the nurse practitioner, there will be such overlap and individuals who work largely in a grey area that straddles nursing and medicine.

King *et al.* (1996) have tried to capture the relationship between advanced nursing roles and medicine in a series of diagrams which are very helpful in visualizing what is happening. Figure 10.1 shows one model of how the area of practice of a doctor and a nurse practitioner may overlap. In this model the nurse enjoys a high degree of autonomy and a scope of practice comparable to the doctor as shown by the circles being

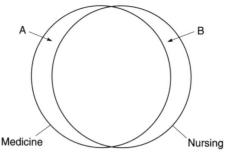

Figure 10.1 Functions of nurse practitioner (NP) and doctor are similar although there are differences such as prescribing powers (A) and health education skills (B). NP enjoys high degree of autonomy, e.g. experienced NP and a GP. (Adapted from King *et al.*, 1996)

equal in size They share much of the same practice with the purely medical crescent (A) perhaps relating to prescribing rights and the nursing crescent (B) concerning health education. Such a model might describe the relationship between a GP and an experienced NP who may become a partner in the practice. Figure 10.2 describes a different model for practice because here the two practitioners still enjoy a large degree of autonomy and extensive scope of practice, but have much less overlap. One example might be the NP working in genitourinary outpatients who supervises and manages a client caseload whom he or she refers back to the GU surgeon only when there are problems which require surgical intervention or specialist investigation. This model could represent a primary care based NP who works on chronic disease management alongside GPs who like to see all first time consultations. In some practices the reverse is the case with the NP taking on the first point of contact role while GPs prefer to concentrate on the long-term management of patients sorting out complex pharmacological problems and monitoring disease progress. An NP-led minor injuries unit might also look like Figure 10.2.

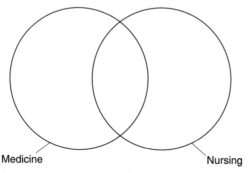

Figure 10.2 Again the NP has a great deal of autonomy but now provides a complementary service to the doctor as his or her function is significantly different, e.g. GU surgeon and an NP working from outpatients to manage patients between surgical interventions. (Adapted from King *et al.*, 1996)

However, Figure 10.3 represents a different situation. Here the nurse is acting as a substitute for a part of the medical role. The smaller circle indicates a reduced scope of practice and less autonomy, while the fact that it is located entirely within the medical circle indicates it is a direct substitution with little or no intrinsic nursing work. Many hard pressed hospital managers coping with the problem of reducing junior doctors' hours may see a nurse and a senior house officer in this way, while some nurses have been developing surgeon's assistant roles along these lines. There is nothing wrong in any of these examples so long as all parties are honest about what they are doing. The nurse is not acting as an NP (see p. 114 for the working definition of an NP) but rather as a nurse specializing in assisting the medical team for the benefit of the patient. This is not illegal or 'unprofessional' in any way. The nurse still needs the necessary education to be safe and effective in the role and the role still needs to be evaluated, however, there is nothing intrinsically wrong here so long as all parties acknowledge what is happening. The nurse is acting in what in America is known as a physician's assistant role. By remaining a nurse, however, this ensures that he or she is bound by the UKCC Code of conduct always to put the patient first, remains within nursing management and education structures and avoids creating a new breed of technician which is the last thing the NHS needs at present. The nurse in this role is probably a cost effective and practical solution to the problem of reduced junior doctors' hours, although that statement is best viewed only as a hypothesis awaiting rigorous research.

It will be many years before expansion in medical student recruitment swells the ranks of junior doctors to levels at which consultants might think that their juniors can cover all the work they have traditionally done, within the confines of a reasonable working week. At that stage will they then say we do not need nurses working in such roles and try to turn the clock back? This is a question any nurse developing a role such as this needs to ask. It is to be hoped that the answer will be 'no, we will not get rid of such new nursing roles', on at least two counts. The first point is the danger of deskilling medicine for, if nurses increasingly take on such roles, the danger is that doctors will find it harder to learn the basic skills

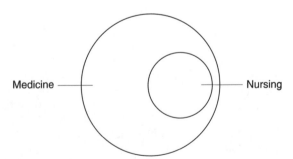

Figure 10.3 The nurse is substituting for part of the medical function hence the smaller circle located within larger medical circle indicating practice within the medical field, e.g. nurse carrying out part of an SHO's role on the wards or working as a surgical assistant in theatre. (Adapted from King *et al.*, 1996)

of their trade. Specialist 'technical nurses' would therefore be a valuable resource in years to come who could teach junior doctors a range of skills and ensure they were performed to a higher standard than perhaps they have been in the past. The second point relates to my argument that the universe of health care is an expanding universe (p. 108) with ever increasing demands. If 6 or 7 years from now, there is a substantial increase in graduates coming out of medical school, then they should be employed more creatively and given better educational opportunities that are relevant to the health needs of the population than they have been in the past. Yesterday's solutions will not tackle tomorrow's problems. In 2005, it is therefore to be hoped that medicine will employ its new graduates in different ways from 1985.

All three of the models outlined above see the relationship between nursing and medicine as very different from the past and of course they only represent three possible positions on an infinitely complex continuum. Many variations are possible and many intermediate positions can occur. All these possibilities are however advocated from the point of view of improving patient services. They all require a recognition that attempting to enforce fixed, definitive boundaries will prevent practice development that is patient focused. They also require educational preparation for the nurse to enable them to function with increased degrees of autonomy and a widening scope of practice (Figures 10.1 and 10.2) or to function in an area of newly acquired skills and responsibilities, possibly under medical direction (Figure 10.3).

Getting others involved in practice development

Having decided that the plans are legal and professionally acceptable, the next question is how do we involve other staff? The first rule is to be as inclusive as possible and to do so in such a way that the possible *implications* of change determine who would be involved just as much as the actual changes themselves. There is a strong view in the literature that this inclusive bottom-up approach holds the key to the successful implementation of change.

The framework within which implementation takes place may be that of a discrete practice development unit (PDU) or a more diffuse practice development network and previous chapters have reviewed the potential advantages that these different approaches bring with them. The importance of recognizing that the whole is greater than the sum of its parts cannot be emphasized enough. Complexity theory teaches us this basic truth, hence the need to try to network practice development as widely as possible and to consider all the possible implications of change as seen from a range of perspectives. We have seen how the appreciation that health care is a dynamic system leads to the recognition that small changes in one place may have major and unforeseen effects elsewhere (a key tenet of chaos theory). This underlines the need for careful evaluation of change which should include the process of change (action research) as much as the outcomes of change. Nurses involved in practice development therefore need to recognize that the only certainty is uncertainty and not be put out by the unexpected. You will never be able to anticipate all the problems. What matters is that any project has good lines of communication so that you find out quickly if there is a problem and you have the authority to deal with problems as they occur. Flexibility and empowerment are essential to enable the project leader to take decisions and ride the roller coaster of change. A bureaucratic, stifling committee structure which takes weeks and months to arrive at any decisions will only lead to the failure of practice development projects as it will never be able to react in time to the unexpected and sometimes unwelcome surprises thrown up by change.

The instruments of change

Preceding chapters contain discussion on the various techniques that can be used such as Lewin's Force Field analysis and strategies for moving change forward. There is compelling evidence in the literature that the successful implementation of practice development depends upon the presence of evidence for change, the context within which change is to occur, and facilitation of the change process. Research projects that investigate the relative importance of these variables are to be greatly welcomed, especially if they explore how they interrelate with each other. The model espoused here looks to have chaotic tendencies, as it is easy to see how variations in one of these three variables could effect the other two in surprising ways.

The model also has to be viewed in terms of time. Practice development can be thought of as the rate of change of practice with time (dp/dt to use the notation of the differential calculus). If practice development is a function of evidence, context and facilitation, does this mean that the rate of change of practice depends upon the rate of change of evidence, context and facilitation? The rate at which evidence is made available and taken up by practitioners, how the culture of a place is changing or how the facilitator becomes known over time, are all examples of how these variables change with time. Theoreticians who would like to work with this model will find themselves straying into chaotic systems and partial differential equations. It is necessary to distinguish between total practice development accomplished over a period of time and the rate at which practice development is occurring. By analogy we distinguish between total distance travelled over a period of time and the rate at which we are travelling (velocity). This therefore introduces a dynamic perspective on the model rather than the static picture which looks backwards at the change accomplished.

Our discussion of memes (Blackmore, 1999) has highlighted a novel way of thinking about resistance to change. It also suggests ways in which we can exploit the characteristics of memes to ensure practice development occurs by the introduction of new memes which will express themselves as changed behaviour. Clinical guidelines may be thought of as memes and to be successful therefore they need:

❏ Fecundity. Therefore they must be spread rapidly which requires a good dissemination strategy and communication networks. It also means they have to have the characteristics of being memorable, making an impact upon the person receiving them and, therefore, being clearly understandable. Above all they have to be seen as useful.

❏ Longevity. Ways must be found of integrating them fully into working practices which will ensure their continuation. This will include feedback on effectiveness and various reminders. Of course we should be careful to ensure that if the guidelines need changing in the future, systems are sufficiently flexible to allow such change to occur.

❏ Copying fidelity. Some variation in implementation between individuals is inevitable, however, the amount of variation needs to be monitored to ensure it does not reach unacceptable levels. We are all familiar with the game of Chinese whispers; a message can easily become distorted if passed by word of mouth only. This emphasizes the need for clear written guidelines and discussion with staff to ensure everybody understands the 'why' as well as the 'how' of clinical guidelines.

A key tool for getting evidence into practice is the systematic review and the York NHS Centre for Reviews and Dissemination plays an important role in producing such reviews on various topics. It is therefore appropriate to conclude this summary by looking at a review they have undertaken on getting evidence into practice. The York Centre (1999) conclude that the following are the key points that indicate likely success in changing practice:

❏ A systematic approach is essential involving strategic planning, i.e. a long-term vision is needed with a clear end game strategy to embed the change in practice or abandon the project if it is seen as not producing beneficial results

❏ All groups possibly affected should be identified and actively involved from the very beginning

❏ The characteristics of the proposed change should be assessed to see how they might influence its adoption, e.g. will this involve nurses taking on traditionally medical work?

❏ The target group of staff involved should be assessed to see how ready and willing they might be to change practice

❏ Potential barriers to change should be identified

❏ Identify likely enabling factors such as skills and resources (this and the preceding point actually consist of a force field analysis)

❏ Dissemination of information in itself will be unlikely to change practice and therefore a broad based, multifaceted approach is needed which targets the different barriers to change in turn
❏ This change must involve personnel who have the necessary skills and knowledge to lead and apply all components of dissemination and implementation strategies (this acknowledges the importance of leadership and facilitation)
❏ There must be evaluation of the effectiveness of change and a structure in place to ensure that the change remains in practice.

This analysis was focused upon medical practice and this should be borne in mind when considering their results. The key finding was that passive dissemination of evidence had no effect upon practice. The York paper for example cites a review of 19 sets of consensus derived guidelines which concluded that there was little if any evidence of any impact upon practice, while a review of 102 studies of interventions aimed at improving health care found a dissemination-only strategy resulted in little or no change. Simply publishing the evidence which supports change therefore is unlikely to have any effect upon medical practice and there is little to suggest that nursing behaves any differently. Mailings, circulars, lectures, published articles in journals are all examples of passive dissemination strategies that have failed.

Introducing an interactive element to changing practice began to show positive effects, however, i.e. where the practitioner received feedback about change. This suggests that active discussion groups might be a better strategy than lectures. Giving clinical staff feedback about change, even if it was merely a regular reminder, was also found to produce a positive effect. The action research methodology advocated here has precisely that effect, unlike the RCT which is the mainstay of much medical research. This suggests that involving staff in change as it happens, rather than carrying out an outcome focused audit at the end, is more likely to produce real change in practise. This view supports the PDU and practice development networking models that are advocated in this book.

Summary

This final chapter has pulled together some of the key themes in this book. Practice development starts by remembering that you are a nurse and nursing is about caring. It has to take place within legal and professional frameworks. Boundaries in nature tend to be blurred and fuzzy areas and so we should not expect things to be any different in the way we, as health care professionals, practise. Practice development cannot occur if we are obsessed with boundaries and defending our nursing turf, instead it happens in precisely those blurred and fuzzy areas that lie at the outer limits of nursing and overlap other professional groups. Whatever the professional territory that we are working in, new nursing roles must be underpinned by education if they are to be safe and effective. While there is not as much research evidence as we might like to guide practice development, there are nevertheless some broad guiding principles in the literature which we may follow with a reasonable expectation of success. The challenge is to work together towards the goal of advancing practice in such a way as to keep pace with the ever changing needs of patients, rather than our own partisan, professional agendas.

References

Blackmore, S. (1999). Meme, myself, I. *New Scientist*, 13 March, 40–44.

King, K., Parrinello, K. and Baggs, J. (1996). Collaboration and advanced nursing practice. In: Hickey, J., Ouimette, R. and Venegoni, S. (eds) *Advanced Practice Nursing*. Philadelphia: Lippincott.

Yeats, W.B. (1893). When you are Old. In: Jeffares, A. N. (ed.)(1990) *W.B.Yeats; Selected Poetry*. London: Pan.

York Centre for NHS Reviews and Dissemination (1999).Getting evidence into practice. *Effective Health Care*, **5**, 1. York: University of York.

Index